T0205527

Clinical Management of Orthodontic Root Resorption

Glenn T. Sameshima
Editor

Clinical Management of Orthodontic Root Resorption

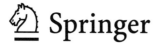 Springer

Editor
Glenn T. Sameshima
Advanced Orthodontics
Herman Ostrow School of Dentistry of the University of Southern California
Los Angeles, CA
USA

ISBN 978-3-030-58708-6   ISBN 978-3-030-58706-2   (eBook)
https://doi.org/10.1007/978-3-030-58706-2

This Springer imprint is published by the registered company Springer Nature Switzerland AG
The registered company address is: Gewerbestrasse 11, 6330 Cham, Switzerland

Contents

Introduction

Glenn T. Sameshima

1   Is Root Resorption a Problem?

One of the most common side effects of orthodontic tooth movement is root resorption, notably apical root resorption, which results in the shortening of the root permanently and is sometimes quite extensive. Although root resorption has been known to occur since teeth were moved and radiographs were available, oddly, this is the first book to devote itself completely to this topic. There is certainly no shortage in the literature; there are well over 1500 articles published of varying types and descriptions at last count.

Clinically, here is the question always posed—is root resorption a problem? The author has heard many times the statement "I practiced for many, many years and never had a problem with root resorption." The cynical answer is that the practice probably never took final x-rays! Root shortening is not a problem until a case gets the attention of the patient or the patient's primary dentist (Fig. 1). Unfortunately, very few dental students are taught anything meaningful at all about orthodontic root resorption in school and learn even less when they got out and practice. Thus, the orthodontist is not only battling his or her own lack of knowledge but that of the uninformed general dentist (or other specialist). For years, it was thought that a tooth with a resorbed root was doomed to be lost, and well-intentioned (hopefully) restorative dentists have told many patients that their short-rooted tooth must be extracted and replaced by an implant. Chapter 9 in this book will explain why this is not true.

The author of this book has spent over 20 years studying root resorption from all aspects: from the cellular/molecular level to large-scale retrospective clinical studies. He has numerous publications on the subject and has lectured to colleagues in both the specialty of orthodontics and general dentistry at many, many international

G. T. Sameshima (✉)
Advanced Orthodontics, Herman Ostrow School of Dentistry of the University of Southern California, Los Angeles, CA, USA
e-mail: sameshim@usc.edu

© Springer Nature Switzerland AG 2021
G. T. Sameshima (ed.), *Clinical Management of Orthodontic Root Resorption*,
https://doi.org/10.1007/978-3-030-58706-2_1

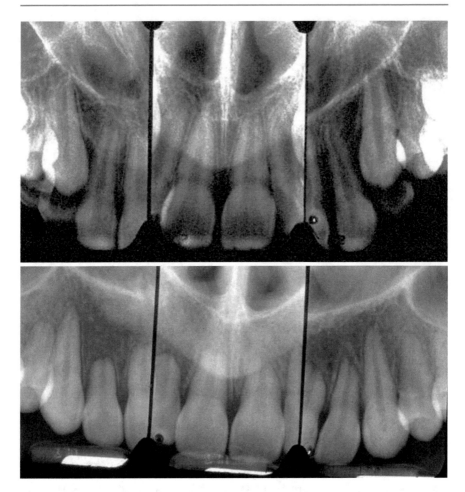

Fig. 1 External apical root resorption—the practitioner wanted to know if he could have prevented the root shortening evident in all four maxillary incisors, what should be done about it now, and if and when the resorption would cease

meetings. He is certified by the American Board of Orthodontics, is tenured faculty at a major US research university, and has 30 years of part time private practice limited to orthodontics. Apical root resorption caused by orthodontic tooth movement is a unique phenomenon and of interest at all levels of clinical practice and scientific investigation.

As is the case unfortunately in many areas of our lives including health care, the specter of litigation, particularly in North America, directs a disproportionate amount of resources to both real and imagined problems brought on by patients and their representatives in the legal business. Orthodontic root resorption is no exception. In fact, in most surveys of the most common legal cases brought to court related to orthodontics, root resorption invariably is found in the top three

Table 1 Orthodontic malpractice claims

- Periodontal problems not diagnosed or not managed before or during orthodontic treatment—21%
- Root resorption as a direct result of orthodontic tooth movement—12%
- Jaw or other types of pain—12%
- Decalcifications and caries—7%
- Other including dissatisfaction with outcomes—31%

(Others include perio-ortho problems, etc.). A quick search of the net using keywords "root resorption," "orthodontic," and "lawsuit" or "legal" brings up some interesting websites. Many of these encourage patients to believe the orthodontist has maimed them terribly, and thus they are entitled to some compensation. Much of what is claimed is not based on facts or evidence, with some going so far as to state that a tooth with a short root is destined to fall out due to lack of support in the jaw. Sadly, there are "expert" witnesses that are more than willing to support the plaintiff in court. Table 1 is based on data presented during the annual session of the American Association of Orthodontists in 2017. Claims of negligence for EARR were 12% of all claims. This number fluctuates every year, but the trend has generally decreased due to the publication of good studies and evidence to refute most claims.

Donald Machen, a real orthodontist and jurist, has kept the profession up to date on legal matters in orthodontics for the past many years. In an excellent article (Machen 2010) about orthodontic ligation, he describes and classifies the various statutes that orthodontic legal problems fall under: paraphrasing—failure to diagnose, which includes unrealistic expectations; failure to respond to the patient's concerns, including failure to treat, failure to refer, and failure to follow-up; and lack of adequate informed consent. Poor, missing, or altered (!) records are more reasons; oddly enough real treatment negligence accounts for only a small percentage of the initiation of litigation. Dr. Machen also emphasizes the need to maintain excellent communication with the patient at all times.

Franklin (2005a, b) discussed the significance of root resorption and malpractice claims. She recommended that the orthodontists monitor the root through "regular radiographs" and inform the patient if once apical shortening is detected. The article emphasized several key points. First, prolonged treatment time is a significant risk factor (see Chap. 5) whether it is from the doctor changing the treatment plan (e.g., waiting to extract teeth) or the patient prolonging treatment through poor cooperation (especially missing appointments). Second, communication is important not just between the orthodontist and the patient/parents but also with the general dentist and other specialists if any are involved in the care. Finally, the need for progress radiographs to document that you monitored the roots is paramount.

In the same issue, a case is described in which severe apical root resorption was found when appliances were removed, 8 years after the initiation of care. The patient missed 52 appointments, and it took 2 years from the time the orthodontist told the patient and their parents the appliances needed to be removed for the patient to finally schedule and keep the debonding appointment. Managing patient cooperation and participation in their own care must be made clear to all parties involved, and this becomes a practice management issue that must be built into office protocols and policies (TDIC 2001).

There are some steps the orthodontist must take to ensure that root resorption is detected during treatment (see Chap. 6). Progress records are important, especially if the patient is at greater risk. It is a known fact that patients who dictate treatment cause treatment to be prolonged particularly if they are constantly demanding that a particular tooth be moved each visit. Imaging at each appointment and periapical radiographs as well as getting a second opinion can mitigate this problem.

References

Franklin E. Losing sleep over malpractice claims. AAO bulletin. Risk management review. St. Louis; 2005a.
Franklin E. Prolonged orthodontic treatment increases exposure to malpractice claims: take steps to reduce risk. AAO bulletin. Risk management review. St. Louis; 2005b.
Machen D. Why are orthodontic lawsuits initiated … and why are the lost. Orthotown. 2010:56–59.
"Resorption. Do your patients appreciate the risk?" Liability Lifeline—published by The Dentists Insurance Company (TDIC) 2001.

Root Resorption

Jing Guo

1 Introduction

Root resorption is a normal psychological process in primary or mixed dentition which results in deciduous teeth exfoliation. By comparison, resorption of permanent dentition, whether idiopathic or iatrogenic, has its similar features histologically. However, it is generally considered pathological and requires the attention of clinical practitioners.

The process of root resorption is attributed to the activity of osteoclasts together with other cells like macrophages and monocytes (Hammarström and Lindskog 1985). Osteoclasts are large multinucleated giant cells associated with the removal and resorption of mineralized bone. These cells are formed by the differentiation of osteoclast precursors (OCPs) generated by hematopoietic stem cells that are originated from the bone marrow (Xing et al. 2005). Osteoclasts can be found directly on the bone surface where resorption happens, or in the Howship's lacuna, a resorption bay at the surface of the bone resulting from osteoclast activity (Hammarström and Lindskog 1985). The equilibrium between bone deposition and resorption is the result of the interaction between osteoblasts, osteoclasts, and their precursors (Márton and Kiss 2014). Cytokines like *receptor activator of nuclear factor kappa B* (NF-κB) ligand (RANKL) and osteoprotegerin (OPG), mainly expressed by osteoblasts and their precursors, are involved in osteoclastogenesis (Abe et al. 2018). RANKL has been shown to be expressed by almost all cell types including endothelial cells, chondrocytes, activated T cells, B cells, and dendritic cells (Xing et al. 2005). The interaction between membrane-bound RANKL and *receptor activator of nuclear factor kappa B* (RANK), its receptor on the osteoclast precursors, results in the differentiation of osteoclast precursors into matured osteoclasts (Abe et al. 2018). OPG is produced by cells of mesenchymal origin and acts as

J. Guo (✉)
Houston, TX, USA
e-mail: guoj@alumni.usc.edu

© Springer Nature Switzerland AG 2021
G. T. Sameshima (ed.), *Clinical Management of Orthodontic Root Resorption*,
https://doi.org/10.1007/978-3-030-58706-2_2

a RANKL decoy receptor to inhibit osteoclastogenesis (Xing et al. 2005). Either RANK in soluble form or OPG can initiate the RANKL-RANK interaction (Márton and Kiss 2014).

External root resorption in permanent teeth is prevented by unmineralized components such as periodontal ligament (PDL), cementoblasts, and precementum (Lindskog and Hammarstrom 1980; Tronstad 1988). PDLs are specialized connective tissues of approximately 200 μm thickness, which attach tooth to the surrounding alveolar bone and serve as a barrier between the bone and cementum (Hammarström and Lindskog 1985). They also possess a protease inhibitory capacity by releasing the anti-invasion factors (AIFs) (Lindskog and Hammarstrom 1980). The hyaline layer of Hopewell-Smith, the intermediate cementum which lies between the cementum and Tomes' granular layer of dentine, seals the peripheral ends of the dentinal tubules and thus can prevent the inflammatory resorption by obstructing the root canal irritant (infected pulp) from the periodontal tissue (Hammarström and Lindskog 1985). Dentine is protected from internal root resorption by odontoblasts and predentin, which together create a barrier against resorption stemming from root canal (Hammarström and Lindskog 1985).

2   Classification of Root Resorption and Causes

Root resorption can be classified by site, etiology, and pathogenesis. In general, the resorption that occurs on the root canal wall is referred to as *internal root resorption*, while the resorption on the root surface facing the alveolar bone is considered as *external root resorption* (Andreasen and Andreasen 1992). External root resorption is further divided into three types: *surface*, *inflammatory*, and *replacement root resorption* by Andreasen (1985). Tronstad categorized the resorptive processes into *inflammatory resorption* and *replacement resorption* based on the etiology and pathogenesis (Tronstad 1988). A summary of the root resorption classification is presented in Table 1.

3   Internal (Root Canal) Root Resorption

Internal resorption is initiated by damage or loss of odontoblast layers and protective predentin and is associated with long lasting pulpal inflammation/infection. Dental trauma, restorative procedures, cracked tooth, pulpitis, orthodontic treatment, and developmental anomaly are the predisposing factors contributing to internal root resorption (Patel et al. 2010). In *transient internal inflammatory root resorption*, pulpal inflammation compromised the integrity of the odontoblasts attached to the root canal wall. As a result, no more predentin is formed in the damaged area (Tronstad 1988). With the elimination of pulpal inflammation, this transient resorptive process can be self-limiting and requires no clinical treatment. In most cases, the loss of intraradicular dentine is permanent and progressive, because the inflammatory processes in the root canal are difficult to be contained. Pulpal

Table 1 Summary of root resorption classification

Inflammatory resorption		Non-inflammatory resorption		
Transient resorption	Progressive resorption	Transient resorption	Progressive resorption	Other
1. Internal inflammatory resorption (intraradicular or apical)	1. Internal inflammatory resorption (intraradicular or apical)	1. Internal resorption	External replacement resorption – *Ankylosis (fusion of the alveolar bone with the root surface)* – *Permanent resorption of dentine and cementum (replacement of bone)*	1. Systemic diseases with dento-alveolar manifestations
2. External inflammatory resorption	2. Internal replacement resorption	2. External resorption (surface resorption)		2. Idiopathic
	3. External inflammatory resorption sustained by – *Mechanical stimulation (trauma)* – *Pressure resorption* – *Infective stimulation (root canal infection)* – *Foreign body stimulation*			
	4. Cervical resorption			

infection is often associated with *internal inflammatory root resorption*; however, microbial stimuli alone do not initiate this resorptive activity. For the progressive resorption to occur, the clastic cells must be recruited and activated. The clastic cells adhere to the mineralized dentin in the resorptive site, where the anti-invasive non-mineralized structures (odontoblasts layer and predentin) are disrupted and the mineralized tissues are resorbed. Therefore, the pulp tissue coronal to the resorptive lesion is usually necrotic, which serves as a source of microorganisms that enter the dentinal tubules. The apical portion of the pulp remains vital, which provides blood supply to the resorptive area and thus a pathway for the clastic cells/precursors to land at the destination (Tronstad 1988). With prolonged pulpal infection, total necrosis of the pulp cuts off the blood supply to the resorptive site completely and thus the internal resorption ceases.

Clinically, *internal inflammatory root resorption* may be asymptomatic in early stages. When the infection occupies the entire root canal and progresses to the extraradicular region, periapical symptoms such as pain on biting may be reported. A classic sign of internal inflammatory resorption taking place in the pulp chamber is called the *Pink tooth of Mummery*, a pink-hued area on the crown of affected tooth (Fig. 1a). Given that *invasive cervical root resorption* (ICRR) may also show a pink discoloration of the involved tooth crown (Fig. 1b–d), ICRR can be often misdiagnosed as *Pink tooth of Mummery*. However, the origins of the resorption of *internal inflammatory root resorption* (from the pulp tissue) and *invasive cervical root resorption* (from periodontal tissue) are different. Clinically, *Pink tooth of Mummery* shows pink discoloration within the clinical crown under the intact enamel (Fig. 1a), while the pink discoloration of an ICRR is from the overgrowth of periodontal tissue that penetrated the enamel (Fig. 1c). The differential diagnosis between these two types of resorptions is critical for early detection and treatment planning.

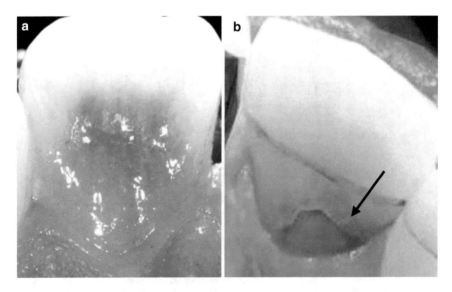

Fig. 1 Clinical photos of internal inflammatory root resorption and invasive cervical root resorption. (**a**) Clinical photo of an internal root canal inflammatory resorption case presenting *Pink tooth of Mummery*. Pink discoloration in the crown of a maxillary central incisor (arrowed). (**b**) Clinical photo of an invasive cervical root resorption. Pink discoloration from the invasion of the periodontal tissue in the crown of a maxillary central incisor (arrowed). (**c**) Radiograph showed cervical root canal resorption. (**d**) CBCT image of the invasive cervical root resorption case which revealed the penetration of the cervical tooth structure (orange arrow), and the invasive resorptive process has extended beyond the coronal third of the root canal (blue arrow). (**a**: *courtesy of Dr. James Simon, Dr. Rafael Roges, and their endodontic residents, University of Southern California, Los Angeles, CA*)

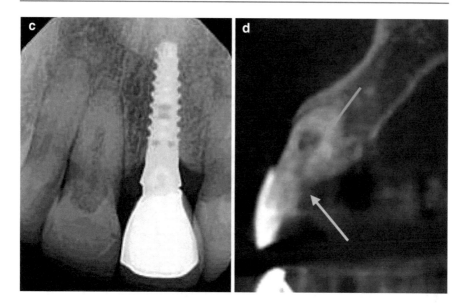

Fig. 1 (continued)

Radiographically, the appearance of the lesion is described as a well-circumscribed, symmetrical, oval, or circular-shaped radiolucency, and the outline of the radiolucency is continuous with the shape of the root canal (Gulabivala and Ng 2014) (Fig. 2). When the resorptive lacunae can be detected by routine radiographs, immediate endodontic treatment is often required to eliminate the source of infection. So that development of fatal result, such as root perforation (Fig. 3), can be effectively prevented.

Internal replacement root resorption happens when the metaplastic hard tissue (bone-like or cementum-like structure) deposits in inflammation tissue after the resorption of intracanal dentine. This type of resorptive defect is associated with low-grade inflammation of the pulp. Histologically, lamellar bone-like structures substituted the resorbed dentine with entrapped osteocyte-like cells (Patel et al. 2010). The origin of the metaplastic tissue may be dental pulp stem cells (DPSCs) which are able to generate reparative dentine-like tissue on the surface of human dentine (Batouli et al. 2003). The mechanism of the subsequent deposition of metaplastic tissue is similar to the formation of reparative tertiary dentine by odontoblast-like cells after the elimination of odontoblasts in pulpal infection. Radiographically, *internal replacement root resorption* displays an irregular enlargement of the root canal space with distortion of the normal root canal outline (Patel et al. 2010) (Fig. 4).

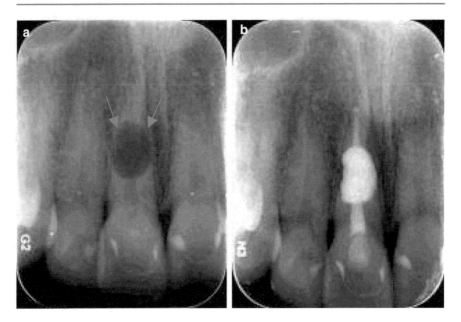

Fig. 2 Internal root canal inflammatory resorption. (**a**) Extensive internal resorption on maxillary central incisor (arrowed). (**b**) Tooth has been root canal treated and obturated with thermoplasticized technique (*Courtesy of Dr. Denny Fang, Irvine, CA*)

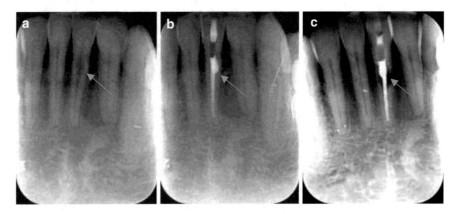

Fig. 3 Unfavorable prognosis of internal root canal inflammatory resorption case failed after root canal treatment. (**a**) Extensive internal resorption on maxillary central incisor (arrowed). (**b**) Tooth has been root canal treated and obturated with thermoplasticized technique (arrowed). (**c**) Resorption continued to develop after root canal treatment and resulted in root perforation (*Courtesy of Dr. Denny Fang, Irvine, CA*)

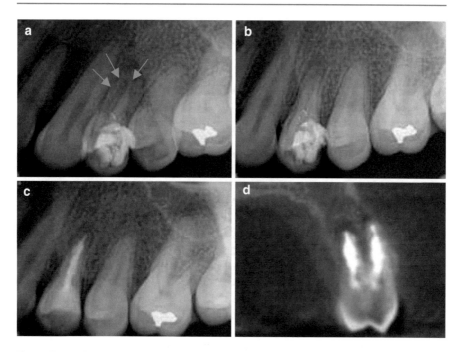

Fig. 4 Internal replacement root resorption. (**a**, **b**) Preoperative radiography of maxillary first premolar with irregular radiolucency in the apical 2/3 of the root canal space (arrowed) with radiopacity appearance inside. (**c**) After root canal treatment with thermoplasticized obturation technique. (**d**) The coronal view of the root canal spaces after endodontic treatment on cone beam computed tomography (CBCT) image

4   External Root Resorption

External root resorption is commonly associated with dental trauma, orthodontic treatment, and periapical periodontitis (Tronstad 1988). Andreasen has classified external root resorption into *surface*, *inflammatory*, and *replacement resorptions*. The location of the external resorption usually involves the apical, lateral, and cervical regions (Andreasen 1985).

4.1   External Surface Resorption

Surface resorption is a self-limiting and transient osteoclastic process followed by cementum healing and reattachment of PDL. It is a consequence of limited injury to the root surface or supporting periodontium, often seen in traumatic injuries and orthodontic treatment (Andreasen 1985). Clinically, *surface resorption* is often asymptomatic and sometimes undetectable on radiographs.

4.2   External Inflammatory Root Resorption

This type of root resorption is caused by persistent inflammation of PDL sustained by mechanical, infective, and pressure stimulation (Tronstad 1988). Clinically, *external inflammatory root resorptions (EIRR)* are commonly seen in patients with traumatic injury, orthodontic treatment, root canal infection, and tooth impaction.

4.2.1   External Inflammatory Root Resorption After Traumatic Injury

EIRR is a severe complication after dental trauma, especially after tooth avulsion. A meta-analysis demonstrated that the occurrence of EIRR in a pooled 1656 avulsed teeth was 23.2% (Souza et al. 2018). An animal study conducted by Andreasen indicated that EIRR can initiate in 1 week after replantation of avulsed tooth in green vervet monkeys (Andreasen and Kristerson 1981). Four prerequisites were proposed by Andreasen for this type of resorption to occur (Andreasen 1985):

1. Injury to PDL, either from mechanical injury from avulsion, laxation, intrusion, and root fracture or from physical (i.e., extending drying time after avulsion) or chemical (improper storage solution, for avulsed tooth) damage of the PDL.
2. Exposure of dentinal tubules of the injured area by damaging the protective cementum/cementoid, in order to ensure osteo-/odontoclastic activity directly on dentine surface.
3. Communication between the exposed dentinal tubules and the necrotic pulp tissue or leucocyte zone harboring bacteria, in order to have bacteria and bacterial endotoxins pass through dentinal tubules to root surface to amplify osteo-/odontoclastic activity.
4. Avulsed tooth is immature or young matured.

Clinically, patient with EIRR may report no symptoms unless the infection becomes acute to show signs and symptoms as acute apical abscess (Heithersay 2007). The radiographical characteristics are a distinctive hollow or blunt surface on the shorten root and a radiolucency in the root surrounding bone (Heithersay 2007) (Fig. 5). Complete cleaning of the root canal system by chemo-mechanical debridement is the key to manage external inflammatory root resorption. Copious irrigation with diluted sodium hypochlorite and long-term intra-appointment medication dressing with calcium hydroxide (Tronstad 1988) are the methods of choice for affected teeth. Calcium hydroxide has been widely used in endodontic treatment as an intracanal medication or an agent for vital pulp therapy due to its antibacterial effect and biocompatibility. Calcium hydroxide is classified as a strong base (pH value around 12.5) and dissociated into calcium and hydroxyl ions in contact with aqueous fluids (Ba-hattab et al. 2016). Its antibacterial effect

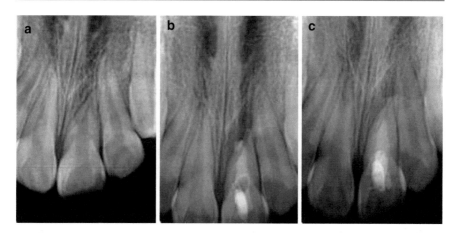

Fig. 5 Radiographs of maxillary central incisor of a 9-year-old boy suffered from luxation. (a) A radiolucency around right central incisor with shortened root. (b) Medicated with calcium hydroxide, extrusion of intracanal dressing was noticed in the periapical region. (c) Extruded calcium hydroxide paste was resorbed by surrounding tissue with reduction of periapical radiolucency. The tooth was obturated with bioceramic material due to extensively enlarged apical constriction by resorptive process

is associated with the high pH value and the ability of releasing hydroxyl ions in aqueous environments. Calcium hydroxide has been playing an important role in treating root resorption since the high pH could neutralize the acidic environment around the resorption site, reduce osteoclast activity, and stimulate therefore repair (Ba-hattab et al. 2016). Heithersay reported a successful trauma case of a maxillary central incisor with external inflammatory root resorption induced by avulsion (Heithersay 2007). The resorption ceased after the application of calcium hydroxide as an intracanal medication over 6 months, and no further resorption has been developed in 20-year follow-up radiographs (Heithersay 2007). However, Andreasen suggested no more than 30-day period of intracanal dressing of calcium hydroxide given to its significantly negative effect on the strength of root, which may increase the change of root fracture (Andreasen et al. 2002). In the 2014 treatment guideline of traumatic dental injury published by American Association of Endodontists, a long-term (2–4 weeks) calcium hydroxide intracanal medication is suggested to prevent rapid inflammatory root resorption of traumatized tooth/teeth if necrotic pulpal tissue has been infected (Trope et al. 1992; Sigurdsson 2014). Moreover, clinicians must keep in mind that the imitation of root canal treatment and the placement of calcium hydroxide should be postponed (about 2 weeks) to allow PDL to heal when treating avulsed teeth with short out-of-socket time (Trope 2002). The rationale is to reduce further damage to PDL caused by the treatment procedure and the necrotization process induced by calcium hydroxide. An immediate placement of calcium hydroxide after reimplantation may increase the risk of ankylosis because of its necrotizing effect on compromised and infected PDL (Trope 2002).

4.2.2 External Inflammatory Root Resorption in Orthodontic Treatment (Pressure)

EIRR sustained by orthodontic treatment, or orthodontic external root resorption (OERR), is an undesirable iatrogenic consequence in orthodontics. The maxillary anterior teeth are the most venerable and commonly affected teeth by OERR (Sameshima and Sinclair 2001a). During orthodontic treatment, the blood flow in the compressed PDL is disturbed, leading to hyalinization of periodontal tissues. The anti-resorptive barrier on the root surface is eliminated by macrophages, and the exposed cementum can be easily accessed and attacked by clastic cells in the favored resorption-promoting environment around a hyalinized area (Rygh 1977). The resorptive process can be arrested when the orthodontic forces are discontinued.

Although most OERR involved teeth remain asymptomatic, the occurrence of moderate and severe resorption would certainly require clinical attention. An estimated 1/3 of the patients who have undergone orthodontic treatment showed more than 3 mm OERR, and 5% of the patients had a resorption more than 5 mm (Killiany 1999). Kalkwarf et al. analyzed the amount of periodontal attachment area lost secondary to apical root resorption in maxillary central incisor models and found out that 3 mm apical resorption was equivalent to 12.9% area of periodontal attachment loss while 5 mm resorption to 26.5% (Kalkwarf et al. 1986). In other words, the initial apical 3 mm resorption was approximately comparable to 1 mm crestal bone loss, and the ratio changed to 2 mm root resorption: 1 mm crestal bone loss when the resorptive process further developed (Kalkwarf et al. 1986).

Understanding the predisposing factors of OERR will facilitate clinicians to precaution potential root resorption during orthodontic treatment. Some of the commonly known predisposing factors include dilacerated and pointed teeth, White or Hispanic ethnicities, and mandibular anterior teeth in adult patients (Sameshima and Sinclair 2001a). With regard to the factors related to orthodontic treatment, a systematic review of 11 randomized clinical trials suggested that OERR is associated with comprehensive orthodontic treatment with heavy forces, especially during intrusive movement (Weltman et al. 2010). Sameshima and Sinclair concluded that first premolar extraction therapy, horizontal displacement more than 1.5 mm, and longer treatment time are significantly associated with OERR (Sameshima and Sinclair 2001b).

Clinically, the involved teeth can maintain vital pulp and remain asymptomatic. Radiographic appearance shows normal PDL space and surrounding alveolar bone, despite shortened root (Fig. 6). Long-term prognosis of OERR is optimistic unless the remaining root length is less than 9 mm in maxillary incisors (Levander and Malmgren 2000).

4.2.3 External Inflammatory Root Resorption Induced by Root Canal Infection

Apical persistent external inflammatory resorption is a complication of root canal infection. Microorganisms and their by-products in the infected and necrotic pulp cause inflammatory reactions in PDL adjacent to the exposed dentine in the apical

Fig. 6 (**a–c**) Progressive external resorption of maxillary anterior teeth in mid- and post-orthodontic treatment (*Courtesy of Dr. Kaifeng Yin, University of Southern California, Los Angeles, CA*)

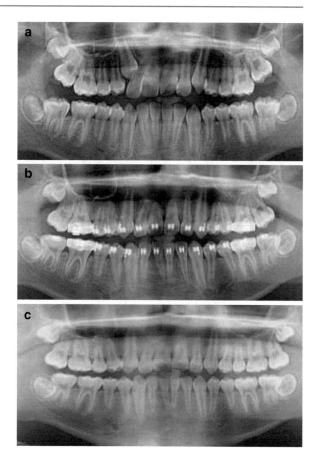

region. Hard tissue resorption stimulators such as macrophage-chemotactic factor, osteoclast-activating factor, and prostaglandins are released to initiate the resorptive process (Tronstad 1988). Clinically, the involved tooth is usually non-responsive to pulpal vitality test. The affected tooth may present signs as symptomatic apical periodontitis or chronic apical abscess. Mobility of tooth may be noticed in case of extensive resorption. A typical sign on radiograph is periapical radiolucency around shortened root of involved tooth. "Extrusion" of root canal filling material can be noticed in unsuccessful endodontic treatment cases due to the resorption of dental tissue in apical portion of the root (Fig. 7).

4.2.4 Orthodontic-Induced External Root Resorption of Endodontically Treated Teeth

Orthodontically treated teeth can be subjected to external root resorption, especially the maxillary anterior teeth (Sameshima and Sinclair 2001a). Compare to vital pulp teeth, whether endodontically treated teeth are more susceptible to orthodontic-induced external root resorption remains controversial. Bender et al. reported one case that orthodontically treated maxillary incisors exhibited severe apical

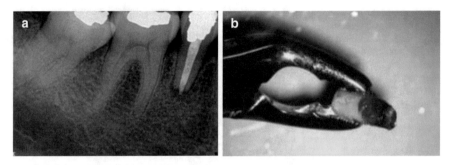

Fig. 7 Apical persistent external inflammatory resorption of mandibular second premolar with unsuccessful endodontic treatment. (**a**) Radiograph shows periapical radiolucency surrounding shortened root with filling material extrusion. (**b**) Photograph after extraction of tooth shows bluntly resorbed root (apex) with gutta-percha remaining extruded

resorption, while little apical resorption was observed in the endodontically treated maxillary central tooth (Bender et al. 1997). The reasons might be the loss of the pulpal immunoreactive neuropeptides due to the removal of pulp tissue during root canal treatment and the application of long-term used calcium hydroxide that can create an alkaline environment in the periapical region (Bender et al. 1997). Other studies have described opposite findings. Iglesias-Linares et al. found that the genetic variations in the interleukin-1b gene (rs1143634) and the genetic variants in allele 1 of the interleukin-1 receptor antagonist gene (rs419598) might predispose root canal treated teeth to external apical root resorption compared to vital pulp teeth (Iglesias-linares et al. 2012a, b, 2013). Recently, A meta-analysis including seven prospective and retrospective controlled clinical trials was conducted, and the result indicated that orthodontic-induced external root resorption was less in endodontically treated teeth compared to their contralateral vital pulp teeth (Alhadainy et al. 2019). So far, all conclusions from existing studies should be interpreted with caution due to the lack of studies in level 1 of evidence. Given to ethical concerns, double-blinded randomized clinical trial might not be applicable at this moment when determining whether endodontic treatment increases the risk of orthodontic-induced external root resorption.

4.3   Invasive Cervical Root Resorption

Invasive cervical root resorption (ICRR) or *external cervical root resorption (ECRR)* is characterized by an aggressively destructive invasion of the cervical region of the root (Heithersay 1999a). It is commonly considered as a subcategory under external inflammatory root resorption. The pathologic process involves a progressive resorption of cementum, enamel, and dentine by fibro-vascular tissues subsequent to the damage to the cervical attachment apparatus below the epithelial attachment. A clinical classification of ICRR has been described by Heithersay based on the extensiveness of the resorption (Heithersay 2004) (Fig. 8).

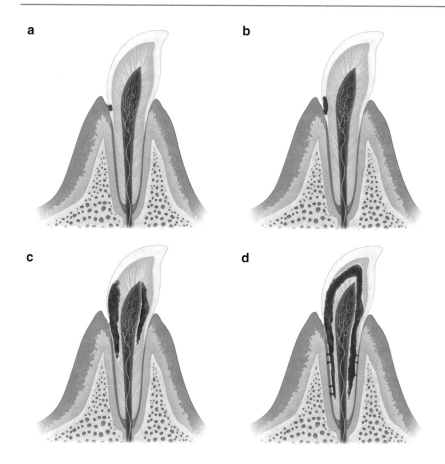

Fig. 8 A clinical classification of *invasive cervical root resorption* by Heithersay (2004) (Adopted from Heithersay (2004)). (**a**) Class I. (**b**) Class II. (**c**) Class III. (**d**) Class IV

1. Class I—a small invasive resorptive lesion with shallow penetration into the dentine near the cervical area
2. Class II—a well-defined resorptive lesion that has penetrated near the coronal pulp chamber but not extended into the radicular dentine
3. Class III—a deeper penetration of resorptive lesion into dentine and extended to the coronal one third of the root canal
4. Class IV—a larger and deeper penetration of invasive resorptive process extended beyond the coronal third of the root canal

The etiology of ICRR remains unclear, and many potential predisposing factors have been suggested. Based on the investigation of 257 teeth displaying invasive cervical resorption in 222 patients, Heithersay assessed 10 potential predisposing factors, including orthodontic treatment, trauma, intracoronal (internal) bleaching,

surgical removal of unerupted or partially erupted teeth or transplantation, periodontal root scaling or planning, bruxism, delayed eruption, developmental defects,
intracoronal restorations, and other potential factors (Heithersay 1999a). Among
all these factors, orthodontic treatment was the most common sole factor (21.2%
of patients and 24.1% of teeth). In patients with orthodontic treatment combined
with other predisposing factors, the occurrence of increased to 26.2% of patients
and 28.4% of teeth examined. The most commonly affected teeth of ICRR after
orthodontic treatment were maxillary canines, maxillary incisors, and mandibular
molars. Potential mechanisms that cause invasive cervical resorption in orthodontically treated teeth are still unclear. One possible mechanism is that the *excessive
forces* during the procedure may cause localized necrosis of periodontal tissue and
initiate the mononuclear precursor cells from the PDL to differentiate into clastic
cells (Heithersay 1999a). Other researchers have proposed the possible correlation
between ICRR and *the amount of tooth movement* during orthodontic treatment
(Dudic et al. 2017). Dudic and colleagues designed a split mouth experiment to
compare the occurrence of cervical resorption on 59 premolars with buccal movement and that of the contralateral control teeth (Dudic et al. 2017). The result showed
that the application of 1 Newton force (around 101 g) over 8 weeks provoked severe
root resorption at the compression cervical sites in teeth with greater movements
(Dudic et al. 2017). Other potential predisposing factors included trauma (14.0%
of patients and 15.1% of teeth) and intracoronal bleaching (4.5% of patients and
3.9% of teeth). In patients with combined treatments (explain combined treatment),
trauma together with other factors constitutes 25.2% of patients and 25.7% of teeth
assessed (Heithersay 1999a).

Clinically, ICRR usually remains asymptomatic unless the pulpal tissue of the
affected tooth is exposed to microorganisms infection (Heithersay 1999b). In early
stages, the lesion displays as a slightly irregular defect at the gingival contour with
soft tissue invasion that bleeds on periodontal probing. Radiographs may or may
not detect the small radiolucency corresponding to this lesion. Histopathological
features of the lesion at this stage usually show fibrous tissue with numerous blood
vessels and clastic resorbing cells adjacent to the dentin surface. Along with fibro-
vascular tissues, fibro-osseous tissues later appear by the deposition of bone-like
calcification onto the resorptive area and within the resorbing tissues (Heithersay
1999b) In a later stage, *pink discoloration* starts to be observed in the crown of
affected tooth due to the cavitation of the enamel overlying the resorptive tissues.
As the resorption develops, the lesion continues to invade the radicular portion of
the tooth, forming resorbing channels into the dentin that surrounds the root canal
space. These channels later interconnect the PDL and extend the lesion more api-
cally. When a more extensive resorption occurs and there is communication between
the resorptive lesion and oral cavity, the invasion of microorganisms starts and thus
triggers the inflammatory response, which is characterized by the infiltration of
acute and chronic inflammation cells in the resorptive area. However, the pulpal
tissue may remain asymptomatic and inflammation-free owing to the protection
of the anti-invasive (predentin) layer (Heithersay 1999b). The pulpal space may

eventually be involved by the invasion of the fibro-vascular tissues if the predentin layer is damaged and no longer serves as an anti-invasive factor (Heithersay 1999a).

ICRR can be often misdiagnosed as a *form internal root resorption* taken place in the pulp chamber, knowing as *Pink tooth of Mummery* (Fig. 1), given that both types of resorptions can show a pink discoloration of the involved tooth crown due to the nature of the invasion of highly vascular tissues (Heithersay 1999b). However, the correct understanding of the origin of the resorption, either an internal one from the pulp tissue or an external one from periodontal tissue, is essential for early detection and intervention of the resorptive process. An accurate diagnosis requires detailed information regarding the clinical signs and symptoms, radiographic appearance, and history of exposure to potential predisposing factors. Conventional periapical radiographs with horizontal parallax technique may be used to differentiate ICRR from *internal root resorption*. When taking two horizontal parallax radiographs of an ICRR lesion, the position of the radiolucency alters when changing the angle of X-ray beam. The radiolucency also follows the SLOB (same lingual opposite buccal) rule and thus is helpful to determine the position of the lesion buccally or lingually. In comparison, an *internal root resorption* stays centered along the shape of the root canal, and the radiolucency does not change its position on angled peri-apical radiographs.

Compared to conventional radiographs, cone beam computed tomography (CBCT) is a novel technique that can provide three-dimensional images with relatively low dose of radiation. With the facilitation of CBCT images, early detection, differential diagnosis between internal and external resorption, identification of the stage of resorption, and treatment planning can be achieved more accurately (Patel and Dawood 2007) (Fig. 9).

The aim of treating the ICRR is to inactivate the resorptive process and to reconstitute the resorptive defect by non-surgical or surgical procedures depending on the severity and accessibility of the resorption (Heithersay 2004). Endodontic treatment may be necessary in both non-surgical and surgical treatments if pulpitis or pulpal necrosis occur. Non-surgical treatment protocol proposed by Heithersay (1999c) includes a topical application of 90% aqueous solution of trichloroacetic acid to the resorptive tissue, a thorough curettage for complete removal the resorptive tissue and the restoration of the defect with glass-ionomer material, composite, or amalgam (Heithersay 2004). Surgical procedure is required when the resorptive lesion is too extensive. A periodontal flap is reflected for the lesion to be accessible, followed by the application of trichloroacetic acid and curettage (Heithersay 2004). The choice of restoration material used in surgical treatment shall be different from that used in the non-surgical approach, because the periodontal reattachment requires the restoration material to provide an effective seal and healing of the periodontal tissue. Mineral trioxide aggregate (MTA) is recommended to repair ICRR surgically because of its superior biocompatibility and sealability (Pace et al. 2008). An alternative to surgical procedure is to apply orthodontic extrusion for better approachability.

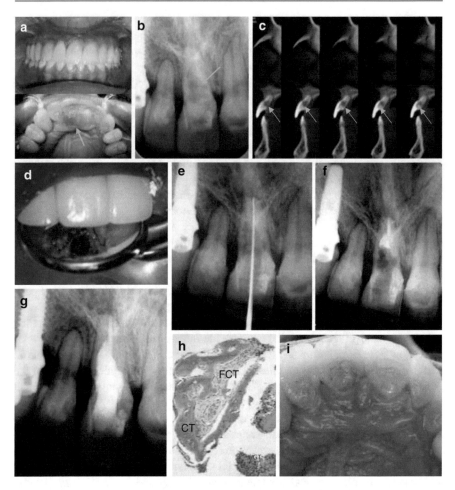

Fig. 9 Invasive cervical root resorption of a maxillary right central incisor with history of trauma and orthodontic treatment. (**a**) Palatal cervical swelling (arrowed). (**b**) Radiograph showed a diffuse radiolucency in cervical area (arrowed). (**c**) CBCT scans showed resorption defects in palatal cervical area associated with periodontal bone loss (arrowed). (**d**) Clinical photo after accessed into the pulp chamber. (**e**) Root canal treatment was performed. (**f**, **g**) Root canal and resorption defect was restored with mineral trioxide aggregate (MTA). (**h**) Histopathological exam of the soft tissue revealed fibroplastic connective tissue (FCT), granulation tissue (GT), and fragments of calcified tissue (CT). (**i**) Postoperative clinical photo after root canal treatment and the perforation defect was repaired (*Courtesy of Dr. James Simon, Dr. Rafael Roges, and their endodontic residents, University of Southern California, Los Angeles, CA*)

Prognosis of ICRR depends heavily on the extensiveness of the resorption. Heithersay followed 94 patients with 101 teeth with ICRR treated with 90% aqueous solution of trichloroacetic acid, curettage, glass-ionomer restoration, and/or endodontic treatment (Heithersay 1999c). The success rates of Class I and II cases were 100%, while 77.8% and 12.5% for Class III and IV, respectively. Therefore, an early detection and meticulous case selection are critical for the prognosis.

4.4   Ankylosis and External Replacement Root Resorption

The most serious types of external resorption are *ankylosis* and *external replacement root resorption (ERRR)*. They occur when extensive necrosis of PDL, and more than 20% of the root surface is involved (Tronstad 1988; Andreasen and Kristerson 1981). The necrosis of PDL can be a result from mechanical injury and physical (i.e., extending drying time after avulsion) or chemical (improper storage solution, for avulsed tooth) damage. Andreasen and Kristerson examined the effect of removing PDL after replantation of incisors in green vervet monkeys and concluded that a loss of 9–16 mm^2 area of PDL resulted in persistent ankylosis (Andreasen and Kristerson 1981).

Occasionally, these two terms are used synonymously. However, *ankylosis* and EFRR are two stages of the resorptive process. There is only loss of PDL and fusion of bone and root surface in ankylosis, while EFRR is characterized as the replacement of cementum and dentine by bone. When *ankylosis* occurs, necrotic PDL loses its viability as a protective layer of root surface. Dentine is exposed following surface resorption, which allows the normal alveolus remodeling process indiscriminately to involve the dentine that is directly approachable to surround bone.

Ankylosis and EFRR are most commonly seen in patients with luxation, intrusion, root fracture, and avulsion injuries (Andreasen and Andreasen 1992). The incidence of external replacement root resorption in avulsion can be as high as 51.0% (Souza et al. 2018). In avulsed cases, extra-oral time greater than 1 h, prolonged splinted time over 10 days, rigid splint, and delayed root canal treatment in matured teeth are all risk factors to ankylosis and ERRR (Von Arx et al. 2001; Kinirons et al. 1999).

Ankylosed teeth can be clinically recognized by the lack of mobility and metallic sound on percussion. Radiographically, disappearing of normal PDL space and fusion of bone and root surface can sometimes be seen in ankylosis, while moth-eaten appearance is typical on root surface with ERRR. In children and adolescents, infraocclusion often accompanies when ankylosis happens, as the adjacent alveolar ridge keeps on developing with the eruption of adjacent teeth (Steiner 1997). When infraocclusion becomes apparent, the ankylosed tooth should be removed, given that a severe vertical defect can happen by retaining such a tooth overtime (Steiner 1997). The time to extract a tooth with external replacement resorption should be the beginning of adolescent growth spurt, usually 10.5–13 years for girls and 12.5–5 years for boys (Darcey and Qualtrough 2013). However, extraction of ankylosed teeth is extremely difficult and often requires surgical procedure. In a worse scenario, the catastrophic loss of ankylosed bone can happen, leading to even more alveolar process defect when considering the nature of thin buccal plate of the maxilla (Malmgren et al. 1984).

A procedure called *decoronation* is a suitable alternative to extraction of teeth with ankylosis and/or ERRR in adolescents (Malmgren et al. 1984). This procedure can completely preserves the alveolar process axially and vertically and thus facilitate the future implant-based restorative plan (Filippi et al. 2001). However, clinicians should not consider this procedure if future orthodontic treatment plan involves space closure of the ankylosed site (Darcey and Qualtrough 2013). This two-phase procedure consists of removing the crown and preserving the root inside the alveolar bone. If the tooth of interest was endodontically treated, all endodontic filling materials in the canal must be removed. Endodontic sealer and filling materials can cause irritation and serve as a potential source of contamination that postpones bone healing. Moreover, the invasion of connective tissue can be seen in a clean and empty root canal, especially when filled with blood, and thus the root can be replaced by bone with time.

Decoronation procedure includes (Malmgren et al. 1984) (Fig. 10):

1. Take preoperative radiographs.
2. Under local anesthesia, reflect a full thickness mucoperiosteal flap buccally.

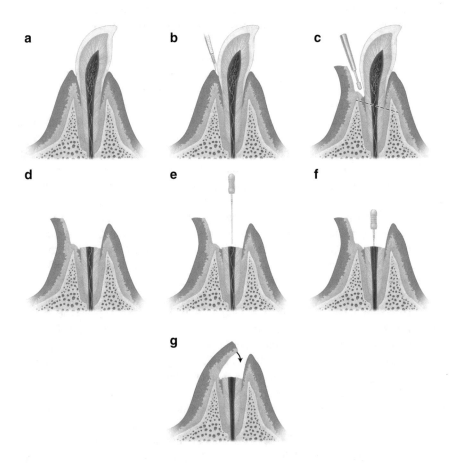

Fig. 10 Decoronation procedure. (**a**) Diagram of tooth with ERRR. (**b**) Reflect a full thickness mucoperiosteal flap buccally. (**c, d**) Cut and smoothen the coronal root surface to a level 1.5–2.0 mm below the edge of the marginal bone with continuous flushing with sterile saline. (**e**) Remove all endodontic materials if needed in the canal, disinfect the canal, and induce blood. (**f**) Fill the entire canal with blood. (**g**) Reposition the mucoperiosteal flap and suture the flap

3. Remove the crown at the enamel-cementum junction using rotary instruments with water spray.
4. Cut and smoothen the coronal root surface to a level 1.5–2.0 mm below the edge of the marginal bone with continuous flushing with sterile saline.
5. Remove all endodontic materials if needed in the canal, disinfect the canal, and induce blood.
6. Fill the entire canal with blood.
7. Reposition the mucoperiosteal flap.
8. Suture the flap.
9. Take postoperative radiographs.
10. Follow up clinically after 1, 3, and 12 weeks and radiographically after 6, 12, and 18 months.

References

Abe T, Sumi K, Kunimatsu R, et al. The effect of mesenchymal stem cells on osteoclast precursor cell differentiation. J Oral Sci. 2018;61(1):30–5. https://doi.org/10.2334/josnusd.17-0315.

Alhadainy HA, Flores-mir C, et al. Orthodontic-induced external root resorption of endodontically treated teeth: a meta-analysis. J Endod. 2019;45(5):483–9. https://doi.org/10.1016/j.joen.2019.02.001.

Andreasen JO. External root resorption: its implication in dental traumatology, paedodontics, periodontics, orthodontics and endodontics. Int Endod J. 1985;18(2):109–18. https://doi.org/10.1111/j.1365-2591.1985.tb00427.x.

Andreasen JO, Andreasen FM. Root resorption following traumatic dental injuries. Proc Finn Dent Soc. 1992;88(Suppl 1):95–114.

Andreasen JO, Kristerson L. The effect of limited drying or removal of the periodontal ligament: periodontal healing after replantation of mature permanent incisors in monkeys. Acta Odontol Scand. 1981;39(1):1–13. https://doi.org/10.3109/00016358109162253.

Andreasen JO, Farik B, Munksgaard EC. Long-term calcium hydroxide as a root canal dressing may increase risk of root fracture. Dent Traumatol. 2002;18:134–7.

Ba-hattab R, Al-jamie M, Aldreib H, Alessa L, Alonazi M. Calcium hydroxide in endodontics: an overview. Open J Stomatol. 2016;6:274–89. https://doi.org/10.4236/ojst.2016.612033.

Batouli S, Miura M, Brahim J, et al. Comparison of stem-cell-mediated osteogenesis and dentinogenesis. J Dent Res. 2003;82(12):976–81. https://doi.org/10.1177/154405910308201208.

Bender IB, Byers MR, Mori K. Periapical replacement resorption of permanent, vital, endodontically treated incisors after orthodontic movement: report of two cases. J Endod. 1997;23(12):768–73.

Darcey J, Qualtrough A. Resorption: part 2. Diagnosis and management. Br Dent J. 2013;214(10):493–509. https://doi.org/10.1038/sj.bdj.2013.482.

Dudic A, Giannopoulou C, Meda P, Montet X, Kiliaridis S. Orthodontically induced cervical root resorption in humans is associated with the amount of tooth movement. Eur J Orthod. 2017;39(5):534–40. https://doi.org/10.1093/ejo/cjw087.

Filippi A, Pohl Y, Von Arx T. Decoronation of an ankylosed tooth for preservation of alveolar bone prior to implant placement. Dent Traumatol. 2001;17(2):93–5. https://doi.org/10.1034/j.1600-9657.2001.017002093.x.

Gulabivala K, Ng YL. Management of tooth resorption. Endod Fourth Ed. 2014:285–298. https://doi.org/10.1016/B978-0-7020-3155-7.00011-4.

Hammarström L, Lindskog S. General morphological aspects of resorption of teeth and alveolar bone. Int Endod J. 1985;18(2):93–108. https://doi.org/10.1111/j.1365-2591.1985.tb00426.x.

Heithersay GS. Invasive cervical resorption: an analysis of potential predisposing factors. Quintessence Int. 1999a;30(2):83–95. http://www.ncbi.nlm.nih.gov/pubmed/10356560.

Heithersay GS. Clinical, radiologic, and histopathologic features of invasive cervical resorption. Quintessence Int. 1999b;30(1):27–37. http://www.ncbi.nlm.nih.gov/pubmed/10323156.

Heithersay G. Treatment of invasive cervical resorption: an analysis of results using topical application of trichloroacetic acid, curettage and restoration. Quintessence Int. 1999c;30:96–110. http://www.quintpub.com.www.libproxy.wvu.edu/journals/qi/fulltext.php?article_id=5310.

Heithersay GS. Invasive cervical resorption. Endod Top. 2004;7(1):73–92. https://doi.org/10.1111/j.1601-1546.2004.00060.x.

Heithersay GS. Management of tooth resorption. Aust Dent J. 2007;52:S105–21. https://doi.org/10.1016/B978-0-7020-3155-7.00011-4.

Iglesias-linares A, Perea E, Solano-reina E. Postorthodontic external root resorption in root-filled teeth is influenced by interleukin-1 b polymorphism. J Endod. 2012a;38(3):283–7. https://doi.org/10.1016/j.joen.2011.12.022.

Iglesias-Linares A, Yañez-Vico RM, Ballesta S, et al. Interleukin 1 gene cluster SNPs (rs1800587, rs1143634) influences post-orthodontic root resorption in endodontic and their contralateral vital control teeth differently. Int Endod J. 2012b;45(11):1018–26. https://doi.org/10.1111/j.1365-2591.2012.02065.x.

Iglesias-Linares A, Yañez-Vico RM, Ballesta-Mudarra S, Ortiz-Ariza E, Mendoza-Mendoza A, Perea-Pérez E, Moreno-Fernández AM, Solano-Reina E. Interleukin 1 receptor antagonist (IL1RN) genetic variations condition post-orthodontic external root resorption in endodontically-treated teeth. Histol Histopathol. 2013;28(6):767–73.

Kalkwarf KL, Krejci RF, Pao YC. Effect of apical root resorption on periodontal support. J Prosthet Dent. 1986;56(3):317–9. https://doi.org/10.1016/0022-3913(86)90011-9.

Killiany DM. Root resorption caused by orthodontic treatment: an evidence-based review of literature. Semin Orthod. 1999;5(2):128–33. https://doi.org/10.1016/S1073-8746(99)80032-2.

Kinirons MJ, Boyd DH, Gregg TA. Inflammatory and replacement resorption in reimplanted permanent incisor teeth: a study of the characteristics of 84 teeth. Dent Traumatol. 1999;15(6):269–72. https://doi.org/10.1111/j.1600-9657.1999.tb00786.x.

Levander E, Malmgren O. Long-term follow-up of maxillary incisors with severe apical root resorption. Eur J Orthod. 2000;22(1):85–92. https://doi.org/10.1093/ejo/22.1.85.

Lindskog S, Hammarstrom L. Evidence in favor of an anti-invasion factor in cementum or periodontal membrane of human teeth. Scand J Dent Res. 1980;88(2):161–3.

Malmgren B, Cvek M, Lundberg M, Frykholm A. Surgical treatment of ankylosed and infrapositioned reimplanted incisors in adolescents. Eur J Oral Sci. 1984;92(5):391–9. https://doi.org/10.1111/j.1600-0722.1984.tb00907.x.

Márton IJ, Kiss C. Overlapping protective and destructive regulatory pathways in apical periodontitis. J Endod. 2014;40(2):155–63. https://doi.org/10.1016/j.joen.2013.10.036.

Pace R, Giuliani V, Pagavino G. Mineral trioxide aggregate as repair material for Furcal perforation: case series. J Endod. 2008;34(9):1130–3. https://doi.org/10.1016/j.joen.2008.05.019.

Patel S, Dawood A. The use of cone beam computed tomography in the management of external cervical resorption lesions. Int Endod J. 2007;40(9):730–7. https://doi.org/10.1111/j.1365-2591.2007.01247.x.

Patel S, Ricucci D, Durak C, Tay F. Internal root resorption: a review. J Endod. 2010;36(7):1107–21. https://doi.org/10.1016/j.joen.2010.03.014.

Rygh P. Root resorption studied by electron microscopy. Angle Orthod. 1977;47(1):1–16.

Sameshima GT, Sinclair PM. Predicting and preventing root resorption: part I. Diagnostic factors. Am J Orthod Dentofac Orthop. 2001a;119(5):505–10. https://doi.org/10.1067/mod.2001.113409.

Sameshima GT, Sinclair PM. Predicting and preventing root resorption: part II. Treatment factors. Am J Orthod Dentofac Orthop. 2001b;119(5):511–5. https://doi.org/10.1067/mod.2001.113410.

Sigurdsson A. The treatment of traumatic dental injuries. American Association of Endodontists; 2014.

Souza BDM, Dutra KL, Kuntze MM, et al. Incidence of root resorption after the replantation of avulsed teeth: a meta-analysis. J Endod. 2018;44(8):1216–27. https://doi.org/10.1016/j.joen.2018.03.002.

Steiner DR. Timing of extraction of ankylosed teeth to maximize ridge development. J Endod. 1997;23(4):242–5.

Tronstad L. Root resorption—etiology, terminology and clinical manifestations. Dent Traumatol. 1988;4(6):241–52. https://doi.org/10.1111/j.1600-9657.1988.tb00642.x.

Trope M. Root resorption due to dental trauma. Endod Top. 2002;1:79–100.

Trope M, Yesilsoy C, Koren L, Moshonov J. Effect of different endodontic treatment protocols on periodontal repair and root resorption of replanted dog teeth. J Endod. 1992;18(10):492–6.

Von Arx T, Filippi A, Buser D. Splinting of traumatized teeth with a new device: TTS (titanium trauma splint). Dent Traumatol. 2001;17(4):180–4. https://doi.org/10.1034/j.1600-9657.2001.170408.x.

Weltman B, Vig KWL, Fields HW, Shanker S, Kaizar EE. Root resorption associated with orthodontic tooth movement: a systematic review. Am J Orthod Dentofac Orthop. 2010;137(4):462–76. https://doi.org/10.1016/j.ajodo.2009.06.021.

Xing L, Schwarz EM, Boyce BF. Osteoclast precursors, RANKL/RANK, and immunology. Immunol Rev. 2005;208:19–29. https://doi.org/10.1111/j.0105-2896.2005.00336.x.

Etiology

Glenn T. Sameshima

1. The etiology of root resorption caused by orthodontic forces is multifactorial and presently not clearly understood despite decades of scholarly activity and publications. Paradoxically, root resorption is common, but clinically significant root resorption is rare. Resorption of the root can occur any time there is injury that produces inflammation in the periodontal ligament or the pulp. As stated in chapter 2, "Root Resorption", classification of root resorption is generally divided into internal resorption and external resorption. Furthermore, there are two types of internal resorption: internal inflammatory resorption and internal replacement resorption. These occur secondary to an insult to the dental pulp and are not related to orthodontic tooth movement. External resorption is classified into four categories: surface resorption, external inflammatory root resorption, replacement resorption, and ankylosis. Surface resorption is the physiologic process of resorption and repair that the root surface sustains during normal physiologic activity (e.g. mastication). External inflammatory root resorption includes any resorption mediated by the inflammatory process and includes resorption caused by orthodontic tooth movement, trauma, etc. This type of resorption can occur anywhere on the root resurface where there is periodontal attachment. Of interest to the orthodontist is the occurrence of external apical root resorption.

2. In normal orthodontic tooth movement, external root resorption is a naturally occurring side effect of the physiological process of resorption and deposition as the bone remodels to accommodate the moving tooth caused by a cascading series of events initiated by pressure and tension in the PDL. On the pressure side of the root, as clastic cells are recruited during the initial inflammatory process, cementoclasts remove cementum—this is normal and has been shown to occur without exception. Along the side of the root, the cementum is repaired as soon as the force expression diminishes and cementoblasts replace the cementoclasts

G. T. Sameshima (✉)
Advanced Orthodontics, Herman Ostrow School of Dentistry of the University of Southern California, Los Angeles, CA, USA
e-mail: sameshim@usc.edu

© Springer Nature Switzerland AG 2021
G. T. Sameshima (ed.), *Clinical Management of Orthodontic Root Resorption*,
https://doi.org/10.1007/978-3-030-58706-2_3

(Fig. 1). This ongoing, cyclic, resorption/repair process along the sides of the root occurs generally without consequence to the health and longevity of the tooth (Fig. 2). Lighter forces generally produce fewer craters on the root surface than heavier forces (Darendeliler et al. 2004). However, in susceptible individuals the normal cycle is disrupted (Fig. 3). Also, for reasons that are not

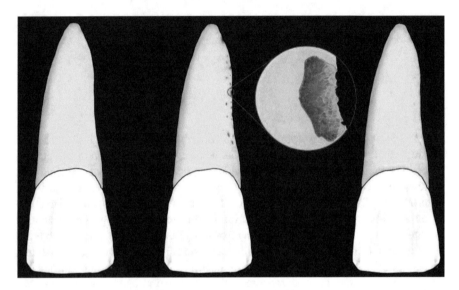

Fig. 1 Cycle of surface resorption. Left: before the application of force—the root surface is smooth. Middle: active tooth movement, pressure side shows damage to surface caused by osteoclasts (brown spots). Enlargement shows the pressure caused "crater" as seen on SEMs of teeth extracted during active tooth movement. Right: forces have dissipated, and the surface repairs itself (faint brown spots represent areas damaged but healing) eventually returning to pre-tooth movement levels

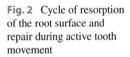

Fig. 2 Cycle of resorption of the root surface and repair during active tooth movement

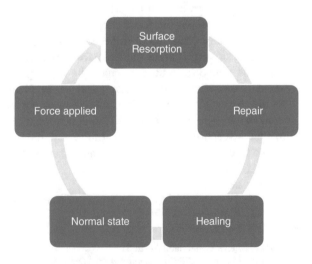

Fig. 3 Cycle of remodeling—unlike the root surface, at the apex of the tooth, the cycle can be interrupted when an unknown combination of factors causes unrepairable damage. This results in permanent and irreversible apical root resorption. If forces are continued and the factors remain, then the cycle repeats, and more apical damage results

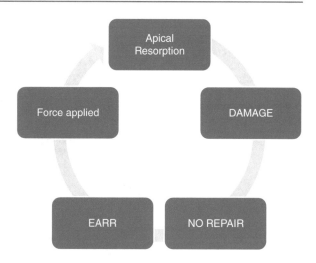

completely understood, the resorption/repair process is different at the apex. Once resorption starts at or near the apex, it does not always repair. The role of exposed dentin may be a factor, or the possible involvement of the pulp through the apices. The apex itself is complex with multiple foramina and complicated surface anatomy. Studies have shown that the composition of cementum is variable near the apex. Stresses on the neurovascular bundle exiting the pulp may be involved. It is important to distinguish between the two forms (location) of external root resorption because what may be true in the former may not necessarily be so for the latter. In order to differentiate the unique type of resorption that takes place at the root apex, the term external apical root resorption (EARR) is the most appropriate nomenclature.

3. Our understanding of the etiology of EARR has evolved over the years. EARR has been the subject of study since the day of Angle and biomechanics was thought to be the main reason. According to Wahl (2005), Albin Oppenheim of Vienna and later, the University of Southern California, wrote about orthodontic root resorption in 1936. Clinically it was observed that there was something about the patient that was the cause, and in the 1950s, 1960s, 1970s, and 1980s, it was generally thought that teenaged female patients were at risk but that was because the vast majority of patients were teenaged females. As the age of genetics dawned, it became evident that patient characteristics were probably genetic or epigenetic in origin, with many cases being due to individual patient susceptibility. In those cases there was nothing to indicate EARR would occur (Sharab et al. 2015). Figures 4 and 5 compare the etiology of EARR in 1980 and 2020.

The role of cementum in root resorption is crucial, but the biology of cementum remains elusive. It is not glamorous or well-funded to study cementum. Most of what we know was published over half a century ago. There are two kinds of cementum: cellular and acellular. Neither seems to play a significant role in *apical* root

Fig. 4 Etiology of root resorption circa 1980. Note that the majority opinion was that something the dentist did with the orthodontic appliances caused the root resorption

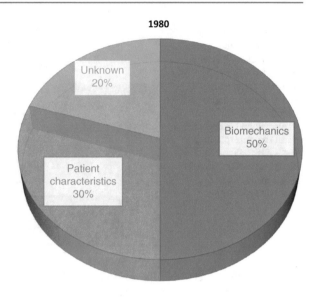

Fig. 5 Etiology of root resorption circa 2020. Rapid advances in genetics and physiology now account for the majority of theoretical causes of root resorption. Note genetics includes most diagnostic risk factors—see chapter "Risk Factors"

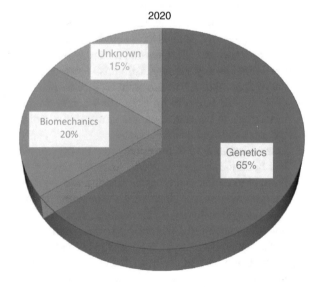

resorption, which again must be emphasized is different from root *surface* resorption. Why? Any dental anatomy textbook will provide the answer. The root apex is a complicated system, not just one clean open apex. There are often numerous foramina, and the apex is never smooth and rounded. Under higher magnification it is possible to observe projections of the apical surface—these could be foci of stress and initiators of irreversible resorption.

A fascinating theory was recently advanced by Brezniak and Wasserstein (2019) whereby as the apex is displaced the hard tissues must "protect" the neurovascular bundle with "irreversible and reversible" mechanisms. As they further explain—despite some of the heavy forces placed on the apex by orthodontic appliances (and also mastication)—teeth never become devitalized. This would also explain the transient pulpalgia often experienced by our patients, especially with initial archwires or trays. And notably, this would also explain why teeth with previous trauma can suddenly become symptomatic when orthodontic forces are applied to them. Furthermore, it is in line with the clinical observation that teeth with immature apices generally do not experience EARR—see next chapter.

In summary of etiology, the physiological "cause" is understood, but why it occurs more readily in some patients and not others is not known. Like most disease states with complex symptomatology but little morbidity and mortality, EARR is epigenetic in origin with layered etiologies which will remain elusive for a considerable time to come.

References

Brezniak N, Wasserstein A. Apical root shortening versus root resorption—is there a difference? Am J Orthod Dentofac Orthop. 2019;156(2):164.

Darendeliler MA, Kharbanda OP, Chan EK, Srivicharnkul P, Rex T, Swain MV, Jones AS, Petocz P. Root resorption and its association with alterations in physical properties, mineral contents and resorption craters in human premolars following application of light and heavy controlled orthodontic forces. Orthod Craniofac Res. 2004;7(2):79–97.

Sharab LY, Morford LA, Dempsey J, Falcão-Alencar G, Mason A, Jacobson E, Kluemper GT, Macri JV, Hartsfield JK Jr. Genetic and treatment-related risk factors associated with external apical root resorption (EARR) concurrent with orthodontia. Orthod Craniofac Res. 2015;18(Suppl 1):71–82.

Wahl N. Orthodontics in 3 millennia. Chapter 4: the professionalization of orthodontics (concluded). Am J Orthod Dentofac Orthop. 2005;128(2):252–7.

Diagnosis

Glenn T. Sameshima

1 Detecting EARR

1.1 Radiographs

Excellent diagnostic images are needed for both diagnosis of EARR (risk factors) and detection of EARR. Modern images provide exponentially more information (see chapter "Imaging"), but the vast majority of practicing dentists in the world today do not use 3D due to the cost and concerns about radiation. In orthodontics, panoramic films are nearly universal, as are periapical radiographs.

Periapical x-rays taken with the beam as close to perpendicular as possible with the roots are the medium of choice due to wide availability and cost. Digital radiographs should be taken for reduced exposure to ionizing radiation and for the environment. For anterior periapicals, the entire root should be visible with good contrast, definition, and high resolution. When viewing the films, the software used should be manipulated to produce the best images, including algorithms to enhance the difference in gray scale layers such that visualizing the periodontal ligament and apex is maximized.

Panoramic radiographs taken on newer digital machines feature low radiation and are far more diagnostic than wet films of yore. They are easily sent among colleagues and if taken properly allow excellent visualization of the teeth, including the roots. According to the study by Sameshima and Asgarifar (2001), periapicals are superior to PANs for the evaluation of EARR, but the study was done on wet films. Periapicals have the advantage of less distortion if the film plane is positioned parallel to the root.

One problem with using PANs is illustrated in Figs. 1 and 2:

G. T. Sameshima (✉)
Advanced Orthodontics, Herman Ostrow School of Dentistry of the University of Southern California, Los Angeles, CA, USA
e-mail: sameshim@usc.edu

© Springer Nature Switzerland AG 2021
G. T. Sameshima (ed.), *Clinical Management of Orthodontic Root Resorption*,
https://doi.org/10.1007/978-3-030-58706-2_4

Fig. 1 Pre- and post-treatment (Phase I) PANs illustrating the effect of proclination and distortion of the PAN on incisor root length

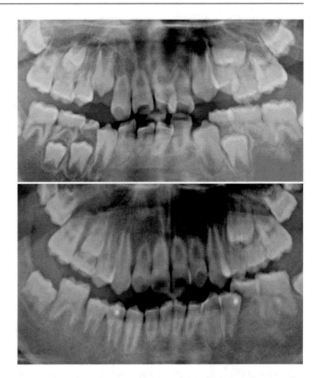

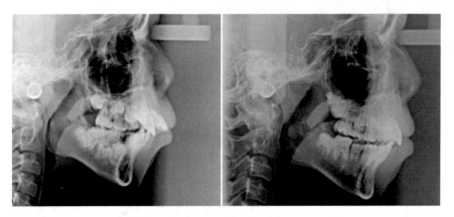

Fig. 2 Pre- and post-treatment (Phase I) cephalometric films showing the change in angulation of the maxillary and mandibular incisors from protrusion to ideal

In the first PAN, the maxillary incisor roots appear to be short and have an abnormal shape. The cephalometric film shows how proclined the incisors are. After Phase I the maxillary incisors are in better position. The roots are still oddly shaped, but their length is less distorted, and they appear much longer. The change is also due to less than desirable positioning of the patient in the initial PAN.

The case shown in Fig. 3 also illustrates the superiority of periapicals compared to PANs in accurately assessing root length and shape. It is very difficult to see the root apex dilacerations of the maxillary lateral incisors on the PAN, and the mandibular incisors are distorted because they are proclined relative to the plane of the PAN machine.

In this next case, the patient was referred by the orthodontist for surgical exposure of the impacted left canine (see Fig. 4 initial PAN). The surgeon advised the patient that the lateral incisor would have to be extracted due to damage from the impacted canine. The orthodontist reviewed the case again with the patient to ensure

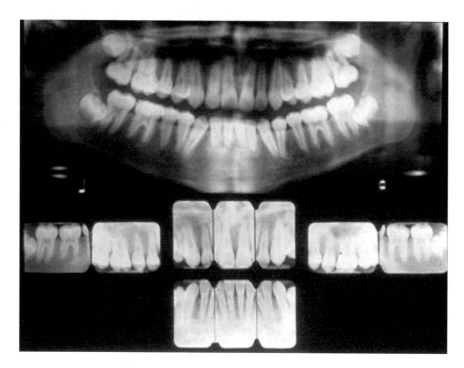

Fig. 3 Pre-treatment PAN, bitewing x-rays, and anterior periapical films

Fig. 4 Initial PAN. The maxillary left canine is erupting ectopically

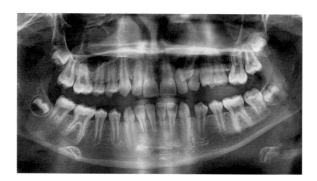

Fig. 5 Magnification of Fig. 4 showing the outline of the root is visible. A 3D scan would have confirmed the normal root length

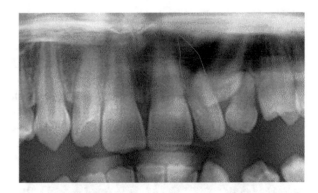

Fig. 6 Progress PAN taken 6 months later, and it is clear that the root of the lateral incisor is undamaged

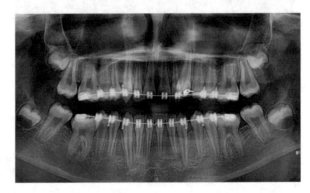

her that the tooth was not damaged. Upon enhancing the PAN (Fig. 5), it is evident the root is undamaged. It was uncovered without incident. The progress PAN (Fig. 6) shows the long dilacerated root of the lateral incisor after the canine was brought into the arch.

1.2 Symptoms

Do patients with active apical root resorption have any clinical signs and symptoms? Do they feel any pain or altered sensation upon mastication or speech? Do they have the signs and symptoms associated with pulpal problems such as temperature sensitivity? Do the teeth discolor? Is there increased tooth mobility? It would be useful if the clinician could tell just based on positive answers to these queries. Unfortunately, the answer to all of these questions is no. There is no pain of any kind associated with ongoing EARR. If there is pulpal insult, it is caused by hyperocclusion or defective restoration or a cracked tooth. Likewise any color change is due to previous trauma and an already damaged pulp. Tooth mobility is not related to root length, but health of the periodontium and teeth are routinely quite mobile off and on during orthodontic tooth movement. However, it would be wise for the clinician to take progress radiographs should the case be going long with apical displacement and notable mobility over an extended time period.

1.3 Other Diagnostic Methods

Limited field cone beam CT-generated volumes can provide very detailed three-dimensional images with the right software – see chapter 6 "Imaging". The field is rapidly evolving with each new generation of both hardware and software using less radiation and producing higher quality images for viewing and manipulating the images in real 3F in real time. They are also far more user-friendly now. There is still no non-ionizing radiation device for routine use in dental imaging.

Gingival crevicular fluid (GCF). Valid attempts have been made to assess markers in saliva or gingival crevicular fluid as non-ionizing methods to detect EARR early in treatment. Several investigators (Mah and Prasad 2004; Balducci et al. 2007; George and Evans 2009) were able to detect levels of dentin phosphoproteins in GCF that were indicative of ongoing resorption. This was found both in primary teeth resorbing naturally and teeth undergoing orthodontic tooth movement. More recently in 2019, a systematic review was published that summarized current knowledge; seven articles that met the standards for inclusion, and the results showed dentine phosphoproteins could be a "potential biomarker," but other moieties, such as dentin sialoprotein, were not (Tarallo et al. 2019). Saliva itself has great potential, assuming there are biomarkers for EARR found in blood-this has been reported in the interesting papers by Ramos Sde et al. (2011) and Yoshizawa et al. (2013).

2 How Is Root Resorption Measured?

Direct measurements on pre- and post-treatment radiographs in millimeters, are subtracted. Some studies standardized periapicals with a custom jig so that both sets of periapicals are taken in the exact same orientation to the crown. There are limitations to this method—tipped teeth are difficult to measure, and the center of the root may be obscured. Most studies measured the distance between the linear center of the incisal edge to the root apex. Another common method is to identify the mesial and distal CEJ and take the midpoint of the line joining the points and measuring the distance from that point to the root apex (Fig. 7). Both methods introduce error, and it is debatable whether any increase in precision or accuracy is obtained by the latter method. Subjective method: the examiner views both pre- and post-treatment radiographs and uses a subjective scale to measure the root shortening. This method can also be used without pre-treatment films but is clearly less accurate. A few published studies used post-treatment radiographs only, and the investigator estimated the amount of root resorption subjectively.

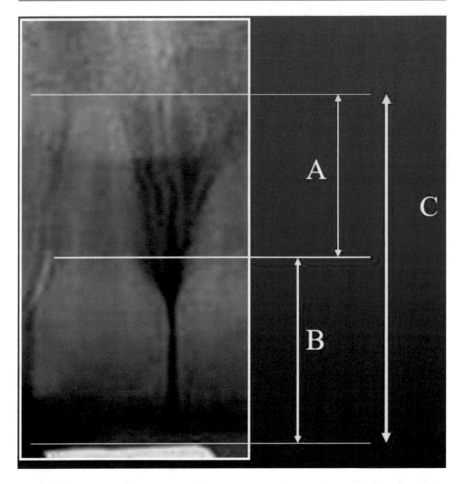

Fig. 7 Common method to measure root resorption from pre- and post-treatment periapical radiographs. It is probably no more accurate than just using the midpoint of the incisal edge to the most apical part of the apex (distance C)

3   What Is Severe Root Resorption?

We learned in chapter "Etiology" that every tooth undergoes surface resorption during orthodontic tooth movement. But are there any teeth that are more at risk than others? The consensus of many, many studies of various populations is that the maxillary incisors are the most affected. Within that group lateral incisors are consistently found to be the most resorbed (Sameshima and Sinclair 2001; Sameshima and Sinclair 2004; Vlaskalic et al. 1998, Brezniak and Wasserstein 2002, Krishnan 2017). Maxillary canines are next, then mandibular canines and incisors. If EARR is found in molars, it is usually the mesial root of the first molar. See Table 1.

Table 1 Mean EARR (adapted from Sameshima and Sinclair 2001)

Anterior teeth: mean root resorption	
Maxillary central incisors	1.27 mm
Maxillary lateral incisors	1.52 mm
Maxillary canines	1.16 mm
Mandibular central incisors	0.69 mm
Mandibular lateral incisors	0.84 mm
Mandibular canines	0.91 mm
Posterior teeth: mean root resorption	
Maxillary first molar	0.11 mm
Maxillary second premolar	0.23 mm
Maxillary first premolar	0.10 mm
Mandibular first molar	0.42 mm
Mandibular second premolar	0.55 mm
Mandibular first premolar	0.37 mm

Table 2 Severity of EARR

Less than 2 mm	Mild or none
2–4 mm	Moderate
>4 mm	Severe

Why maxillary lateral incisors? They have the highest frequency of dilaceration of all the teeth. Because of their pivotal position in the arch, the "Social Six" the root apex is moved in all three planes of space much more than the rest of the dentition. Maxillary lateral incisors also have a high occurrence rate of peg shape, barrel shape, and other odd features. Chapter 9 "Resorption of Impacted Teeth" will discuss lateral incisors in the context of the eruption of the maxillary canine, and it will be shown that the root is often damaged.

The mean (average) EARR of maxillary incisors (most resorbed teeth) found in the literature is approx. 1.2–1.4 mm. There are no consensus standards on what constitutes severe EARR. In a paper by Lee et al. (2003), general dentists said 35% root shortening should terminate orthodontic treatment; orthodontists surveyed were less conservative, meaning they allowed slightly more EARR before stopping treatment.

Generally for a normal length, non-periodontally involved tooth, the following ranges are defined by convention (Table 2 and Fig. 8):

For example Brin et al. (2003) found that 11% of central and 14% of lateral incisors demonstrated moderate to severe (>2 mm) EARR. Sameshima and Sinclair (2004) published similar findings.

Surface area of a root and severity: the loss of a third of a root generally translates into a loss of a third of its surface area, assuming the apical third is a paraboloid and the coronal two-thirds are cylindrical. However, if we assume that the entire root is a paraboloid, then the root surface loss is only 23%. For EARR of 50%, the surface area is reduced by 39%. For EARR of two-thirds of the original root length, the surface area reduction is 57%. If two teeth have the same root shape but one is twice as long as the other, then the shorter tooth will have 62% less surface area, not 50%. Surface area is important in the long run because it establishes the number of fibers in the PDL that secure the root to the bone.

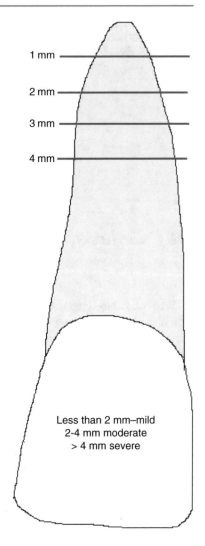

Fig. 8 Maxillary central incisor—EARR severity based on millimeters of root lost on a periapical x-ray

4 Short Root Anomaly

4.1 Diagnosis of Short Root Anomaly

Can I move teeth with really short roots? There is no evidence that teeth with short roots are at higher risk. One study found a positive association between amount of EARR and root length, but this has not been confirmed by other studies. Short roots are not higher risk, but the consequences should EARR occur are obviously of much greater concern. One or two teeth can be short from a history of trauma, but essentially multiple short rooted teeth are genetically inherited.

It is vitally important to distinguish a patient with one or two teeth with relatively short roots, from a patient who has "short root anomaly." This is a documented condition that must be recognized by every dentist. Short root anomaly (SRA) was given this name by Volmer Lind in 1972. He defined SRA as "abnormally short, plump roots always affecting the maxillary central incisors and rarely any other teeth (Lind, 1972)." The prevalence in a northern European population was reported to be 1.3% in 2000 students by Apajalahti et al. (2002). They defined SRA as maxillary central incisors with a crown to root ratio greater than or equal to one. SRA is considered a familial condition (Apajalahti et al. 1999). And although the specific inheritance pattern and gene families have not been identified, a thesis by Nayak (2018) demonstrated a link between the interleukin family and SRA. Nayak studied a cohort of 26 patients with SRA matched to 26 patients without SRA. Using genomic DNA samples, she found that all of the patients in the SRA group exhibited the CC genotype for the IL-1β gene polymorphism at +3954. This genotype has been implicated in causing increased root. They also found that Hispanic patients were significantly more prevalent in the SRA group and had the same genotype +3954. They concluded that Hispanic patients may be at a higher risk for orthodontically induced root resorption due to this genotype (See ethnicity risk factors in next chapter.) Puranik et al. (2015) had also reported a higher prevalence of SRA in Hispanic subjects; this has been observed clinically for many years in communities with large Hispanic populations. The question of significance in the Hispanic population may be tempered by the findings of Wang et al. (2019) that showed that this group had a significantly smaller crown to ratio compared to other ethnic groups overall. Prevalence in Asian patients has not been studied but seems to be higher than in Caucasians. The literature can be confusing as the distinction between idiopathic root resorption, SRA, and persons who just have short roots (or syndromes) is often blurred.

Is SRA a risk factor for EARR? It has historically been suspected, even assumed due to the odd root shape that SRA central incisors usually have. Lind wrote that SRA had higher EARR in 1972. However, the study by Cutrera et al. (2019) at UConn showed no difference between 23 SRA patients and 26 control patients using pre- and post-treatment CBCT scans.

4.2   Summary of SRA

1. A patient with maxillary central incisors with short, possibly blunted roots may have short root anomaly. Other teeth, most commonly second bicuspids, are also affected and appear shorter than normal on radiographs.
2. It is important to differentiate between SRA and idiopathic root resorption. The latter is a true apical resorption; the former is congenitally short roots.
3. The study at UConn seems to show there is no greater risk for EARR for patients with SRA of the maxillary central incisors. Further studies are needed.
4. There is evidence that SRA is much more common in Hispanic patients.

Clinical Case 1

Age 10.1 female at start of orthodontic treatment for minor crowding and rotations. Maxillary protrusion treated with first bicuspid extractions and fixed appliances for 2 years. The crown to root ratio of the maxillary central incisors is slightly less than one. The second bicuspids are not fully developed, but even at this stage, they are short. See Figs. 9 and 10.

Clinical Case 2 See Fig. 11 Initial PAN

Hispanic 10-year-old male. Negative health history. No history of trauma. CC: crowding, "fang teeth." Dentoalveolar protrusion by all ceph numbers. Normal overjet but deep (50%) bite. Treatment plan: extract first bicuspids, fixed appliances 0.018 SWA.

Fig. 9 Initial PAN

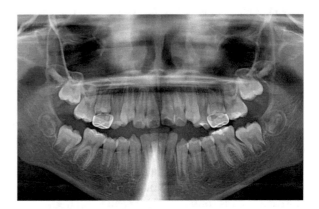

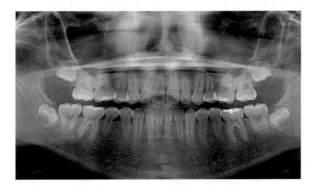

Fig. 10 Final PAN after 20 months of treatment with 0.022 SWA. Finishing elastics were prescribed for a short period. Minimum anchorage. Very minor rounding of the apices of the maxillary incisors can be observed. The second bicuspid roots are short. Was this a case of short root anomaly? The central incisors were marginally short, and the patient was a Hispanic female

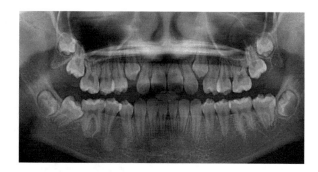

Fig. 11 Initial PAN—note short bicuspids and extremely short maxillary central and lateral incisors. The central incisor roots are pointed. Condensing osteitis can be seen on the mandibular second and first bicuspids. This case would be diagnosed as short root anomaly

Clinical Case 3

Hispanic female age 12 chief complaint is "I have ugly teeth." No previous orthodontic treatment. Had history of allergies; is a mouth breather. Forward tongue posture. Denies habits.

Clinical: skeletal dental anterior open bite with crowding and poor facial esthetics. Oral hygiene is poor. She has moderate maxillary crowding and a bilateral posterior cross bite in CR with a narrow maxilla (Figs. 12 and 13). The pre-treatment PAN shows radiographic signs commonly associated with SRA.

Case 4

10-year-old Hispanic female patient referred by her general dentist for an impacted right maxillary canine. See Fig. 14. From the initial PAN, the diagnosis of SRA can be made based on her short maxillary central incisors. Root formation for all 4 s bicuspids is incomplete; however, it would appear that they will be short as well.

Case 5

SRA. The patient was a 22-year-old Hispanic female. Class II malocclusion with crowding, deep bite, and excess overjet. The maxillary central incisors, maxillary bicuspids, and mandibular second bicuspids are short. The maxillary right lateral incisor root has been resorbed by the erupting canine (Figs. 15 and 16).

5   EARR and Periodontal Disease

There is no direct relationship between apical root resorption from orthodontic tooth movement and a history of periodontitis. Significant vertical bone loss will alter the center of resistance of the tooth, but other factors discussed in the next chapter explain more of the risk. Poor oral hygiene is suspected of being a factor that is not necessary for EARR but certainly does not help.

Case 6 Periodontitis and EARR (Figs. 17 and 18)

26-year-old adult case (Class II) with no other risk factors. All four first bicuspids were extracted for crowding and dentoalveolar protrusion. Total treatment time was

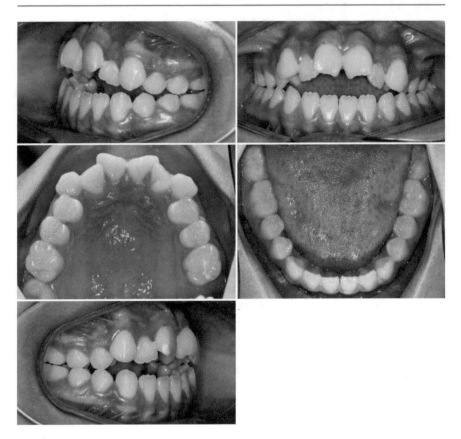

Fig. 12 Initial intraoral images of Clinical Case 3

Fig. 13 Initial PAN This is clearly a case of short root anomaly. Is the patient at greater risk? There are some risk factors for EARR: Hispanic ethnicity, abnormal root shape, and Le Fort I surgery. Is SRA alone a risk factor?

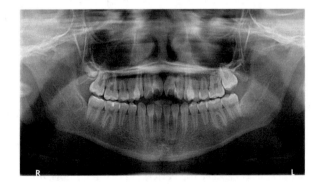

Fig. 14 Initial PAN for Case 4 SRA

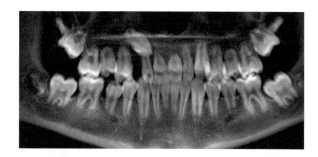

Fig. 15 Initial PAN for Case 5

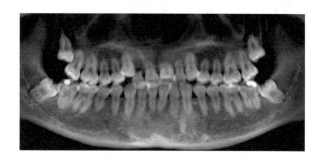

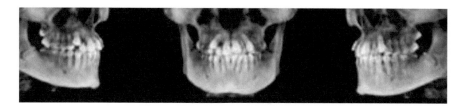

Fig. 16 Cone beam CT scan for Case 5

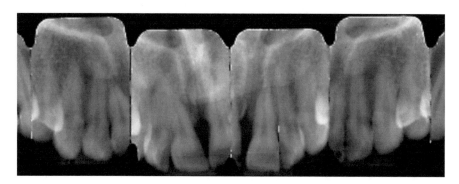

Fig. 17 Pre-treatment periapical x-rays

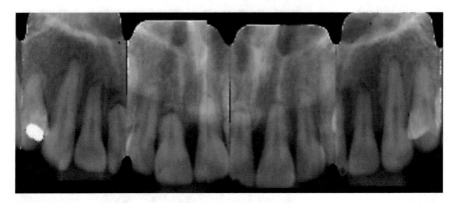

Fig. 18 Post-treatment periapical x-rays

28 months. Fixed appliances were used. Pre-treatment there was a periodontal defect between the maxillary central incisors that had been treated 8 years previously. Post-treatment the right maxillary central incisor had 4 mm of EARR, and the left had 1 mm of EARR, but the vertical bone loss worsened. There was no tooth mobility. Dr. Robert Boyd, chair of orthodontics at the University of Pacific and a board certified periodontist and orthodontist, once said "1 mm of vertical bone loss (due to periodontal disease) is worse than 3 mm of apical root resorption."

References

Apajalahti S, Arte S, Pirinen S. Short root anomaly in families and its association with other dental anomalies. Eur J Oral Sci. 1999;107(2):97–101.

Apajalahti S, Hölttä P, Turtola L, Pirinen S. Prevalence of short-root anomaly in healthy young adults. Acta Odontol Scand. 2002;60(1):56–9.

Balducci L, Ramachandran A, Hao J, Narayanan K, Evans C, George A. Biological markers for evaluation of root resorption. Arch Oral Biol. 2007;52(3):203–8.

Brezniak N, Wasserstein A. Orthodontically induced inflammatory root resorption. Part I: the clinical aspects. Angle Orthod. 2002;72(2):180–4.

Brin I, Tulloch JF, Koroluk L, Philips C. External apical root resorption in class II malocclusion: a retrospective review of 1- versus 2-phase treatment. Am J Orthod Dentofac Orthop. 2003;124(2):151–6.

Cutrera A, Allareddy V, Azami N, Nanda R, Uribe F. Is short root anomaly (SRA) a risk factor for increased external apical root resorption in orthodontic patients? A retrospective case control study using cone beam computerized tomography. Orthod Craniofac Res. 2019;22(1):32–7.

George A, Evans C. Detection of root resorption using dentin and bone markers. Orthod Craniofac Res. 2009;12:229–35.

Krishnan V. Root resorption with orthodontic mechanics: pertinent areas revisited. Aust Dent J. 2017;62(Suppl 1):71–7.

Kook S. Lee, Sorin R. Straja, Orhan C. Tuncay. Perceived long-term prognosis of teeth with orthodontically resorbed roots. Orthodontics & Craniofacial Research. 2003;6(3):177–191

Lind V. Short root anomaly. Scand J Dent Res. 1972;80(2):85–93.

Mah J, Prasad N. Dentine phosphoproteins in gingival crevicular fluid during root resorption. Eur J Orthod. 2004;26:25–30.

Nayak SC. Interleukin-1 beta (IL-B) gene polymorphisms in pre-treatment orthodontic patients exhibiting short root anomaly (SRA). Thesis UNLV; 2018.

Puranik CP, Hill A, Henderson Jeffries K, Harrell SN, Taylor RW, Frazier-Bowers SA. Characterization of short root anomaly in a Mexican cohort—hereditary idiopathic root malformation. Orthod Craniofac Res. 2015;18(Suppl 1):62–70.

Ramos Sde P, Ortolan GO, Dos Santos LM, Tobouti PL, Hidalgo MM, Consolaro A, Itano EN. Anti-dentine antibodies with root resorption during orthodontic treatment. Eur J Orthod. 2011;33(5):584–91.

Sameshima GT, Asgarifar KO. Assessment of root resorption and root shape: periapical vs panoramic films. Angle Orthod. 2001;71(3):185–9.

Sameshima GT, Sinclair PM. Predicting and preventing root resorption: part I. Diagnostic factors. Am J Orthod Dentofac Orthop. 2001;119(5):505–10.

Sameshima GT, Sinclair PM. Characteristics of patients with severe root resorption. Orthod Craniofac Res. 2004;7(2):108–14.

Tarallo F, Chimenti C, Paiella G, Cordaro M, Tepedino M. Biomarkers in the gingival crevicular fluid used to detect root resorption in patients undergoing orthodontic treatment: a systematic review. Orthod Craniofac Res. 2019;22(4):236–47.

Vlaskalic V, Boyd RL, Baumrind S. Etiology and sequelae of root resorption. Semin Orthod. 1998;4:124–31.

Wang J, Rousso C, Christensen B, Li P, Kau CH, Lamani E. Ethnic differences in the root to crown ratios of the permanent dentition. Orthod Craniofac Res. 2019;22(2):99–104.

Yoshizawa JM, Schafer CA, Schafer JJ, Farrell JJ, Paster BJ, Wong DT. Salivary biomarkers: toward future clinical and diagnostic utilities. Clin Microbiol Rev. 2013;26(4):781–91.

Risk Factors

Glenn T. Sameshima

1 Introduction

The busy clinician would like to know if there are any factors that they can use to (1) identify the patient at higher risk, (2) prevent or mitigate EARR, and (3) inform the patient. Commonly EARR is discovered post-treatment (Fig. 1). This chapter will present a practical summary of our current knowledge to help answer the first query—identifying the patient at higher risk. This discussion will be evidence-based but will also include cases and opinions based on years of clinical experience gathered from many clinicians around the world. Table 1 is a summary of factors that will be considered in this chapter.

2 Diagnostic Risk Factors

2.1 Family History of EARR

In chapter "Etiology" we saw that genetics plays a large role in the etiology of EARR. But how does this translate into clinical practice? We have not identified a specific gene or group of genes and even if we did, how would we reliably test for this? The value of genetics in EARR is simple—if you treat a family member and they get a lot of EARR, then the chances that a sibling will get it are much higher than in an unaffected family. Risk is also increased if a *parent* reports that when they "had braces my roots got short."

G. T. Sameshima (✉)
Advanced Orthodontics, Herman Ostrow School of Dentistry of the University of Southern California, Los Angeles, CA, USA
e-mail: sameshim@usc.edu

© Springer Nature Switzerland AG 2021
G. T. Sameshima (ed.), *Clinical Management of Orthodontic Root Resorption*,
https://doi.org/10.1007/978-3-030-58706-2_5

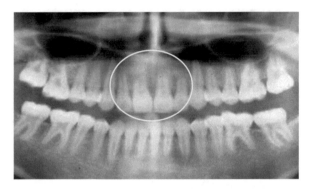

Fig. 1 This is the post-treatment PAN after 20 months of non-extraction treatment with a fixed straight-wire appliance. The clinician asked if there were any factors they might have known or observed before treatment that would have prevented the observed moderate to severe EARR (50% of root length on three of the maxillary incisors) from occurring

Table 1 EARR risk factors

Diagnostic
1. Family History of EARR
2. Positive medical history for known conditions
3. Abnormal root shape
4. Vertical problems
5. Excess overjet
6. Hispanic Ethnicity

Treatment risk actors
1. Apical Displacement
2. Prolonged treatment time
3. Extraction cases
4. Absolute intrusion
5. Heavy forces

Suspected risk factors
1. Maxillofacial surgery cases
2. Impacted teeth
3. Heavy Torque

No Evidence of Increased or decreased risk
1. Malocclusion type
2. Appliance type
3. Slot size
4. Archwires
5. Habits
6. Transverse expansion (unless you run)
7. Hawley retainers
8. Clear aligners
9. Accelerated orthodontics

2.2   Positive Medical History for Known Conditions

Patients who have a history of endocrine problems may have a higher risk although there is not enough solid evidence in the literature to support this statement. Theoretically any condition that would adversely affect tooth movement either directly or indirectly would have an effect.

1. Thyroid and other endocrine problems—there are isolated case reports and communications suggesting this could increase risk. Clinicians should be aware that most endocrine problems and their treatments can affect the biology of tooth movement.
2. Diseases of hard and connective tissue. Patients who are taking heavy doses of anti-inflammatories or anti-osteoporotic medications have resistance to normal tooth movement. These patients should not be undergoing orthodontic treatment, but if they did there might be less EARR due to lack of apical movement or more EARR if unsuspecting clinicians were to apply more force in response to the lack of movement.
3. Turner syndrome—case reports and some evidence for higher risk—there are some reports of EARR with no dental treatment. Patients often have congenitally short roots. EARR is listed as a possible dental side effect on their advocacy webpage (https://www.turnersyndrome.org/dentistryandorthodontics).
4. Asthma and allergies—although there is a reasonable physiological basis in linking asthma with EARR, conflicting evidence exists for asthma as a risk factor (Nishioka et al. 2006; Davidovitch et al. 2000; McNab et al. 1999). Likewise there is no clear evidence either way for allergies as a risk factor (Owman-Moll and Kurol 2000; Murata et al. 2013).
5. Idiopathic root resorption—there are isolated case reports of individuals and families who for no known reason get severe apical root resorption spontaneously, with no association with dental or orthodontic treatment (Rivera and Walton 1994). In some of the case reports, it is difficult to determine if the patient has congenitally short roots or in fact the roots actually resorbed.
6. Familial dysostosis (familial expansile osteolysis)—a rare syndrome affecting bone in which most affected individuals all have severe root resorption (see Mitchell et al. 1990).

There is no clear evidence for habits like tongue thrusting, nail biting, or bruxing as independent risk factors; more likely they are cofactors with apical displacement and long treatment time (Sameshima and Sinclair 2001a, b).

2.3   Root Shape and Length

Figure 2 shows the classification of root shape in 2D. Dental roots that have a shape that deviates from a typical conical shape seem to be at higher risk for EARR. This has been shown by clinical (Sameshima and Sinclair 2001a, b; Brin et al. 2003, many others) and theoretical (finite element) investigations (Shaw et al. 2004; Kamble et al. 2012). Dilacerated, pointed roots, and pipette-shaped roots have a higher risk for EARR (Sameshima and Sinclair 2001a, b). Figure 3 illustrates the typical pattern of EARR for a dilacerated root—note how the dilacerated portion is resorbed. Dilacerated roots are especially vulnerable which double the risk (Fernandes et al. 2019). Teeth with a history of trauma may be at risk, but teeth with prior resorption are not (Brin et al. 1991; Kindelan et al. 2008).

Clinical Case 1 EARR on the Dilacerated Portion of the Root (Figs. 4 and 5).
15-year-old Caucasian male extraction case for crowding, rotations, excess overjet and deep bite, flared maxillary incisors, and poor facial esthetics. Negative health history for EARR risk factors. Orthodontic treatment: 2 years in fixed 0.022 SWA with extraction of both maxillary first bicuspids.

Clinical Case 2 "Wild Dilaceration" but no EARR (Fig. 6)
The patient had unusual dilaceration of both maxillary central incisors; the dilaceration is midway between the root apex and the CEJ (Figs. 7 and 8). There was no EARR at the end of fixed treatment of 18 months duration.

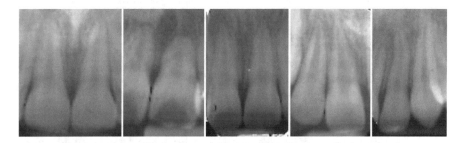

Fig. 2 Classification of central incisor root shape from periapical x-rays (adapted from Sameshima and Sinclair 2001a, b). The classification is also valid for all incisors and canines. From left to right: normal blunt bottle (or pipette) pointed dilacerated

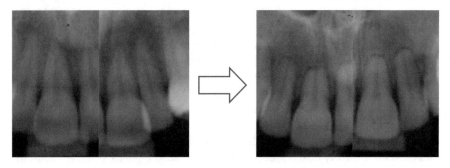

Fig. 3 Typical pattern of EARR when the roots are dilacerated

Fig. 4 Initial
PAN. Dilacerated apical
fourth on both maxillary
lateral incisors. Midroot
dilaceration on the
maxillary left central
incisor. Additional
dilacerations can be seen
on the mandibular
bicuspids and canines

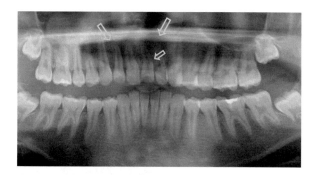

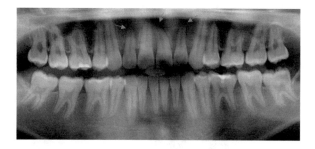

Fig. 5 Final PAN. There is a generalized rounding of most of the root apices of all teeth. Note in particular the lost dilacerated apical portions that were seen pretreatment (see previous figure for comparison). The root apices of the maxillary incisors were displaced bodily, and palatal movement horizontally was 2 mm. Fortunately, the amount of EARR is low; less than 2 mm

Fig. 6 Pretreatment
intraoral image—front.
Note tipped central
incisors, rotated lateral
incisor, and low frenum in
the maxillary
anterior segment

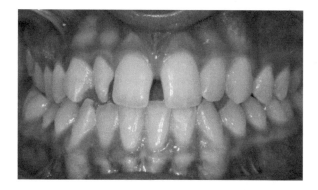

Peg, barrel-shaped, or small lateral incisors – do not have higher risk for EARR according to a split-mouth investigation (Kook et al. 2003).

Tooth Length: Sameshima and Sinclair (2001a, b) found that the amount of EARR correlated significantly with increasing root length. Mirabella and Artun (1995) also found more EARR with longer roots. The lateral incisors were 54% more likely to develop EARR for each additional millimeter of length, and the risk

Fig. 7 Pretreatment PAN of the same patient. Note odd root dilaceration of both maxillary central incisors. This is most likely genetic and not acquired

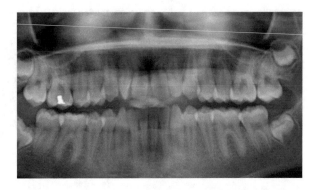

Fig. 8 Final PAN. There is no change in root length (difficult to see the left incisors due to the artifact)

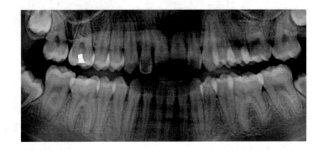

of EARR increased by 29% in the paper by Fernandes et al. (2019). Thus, clinically, short-rooted teeth per se are not at higher risk and may have <u>less</u> risk.

2.4 Vertical Problems

Historically both open and deep bites were associated with increased risk for EARR (Harris and Butler 1992, Sameshima and Sinclair 2001a, Zhou 2015), however, the magnitude and direction of apical displacement may be the primary factor.

An interesting thesis investigated the outcomes of the MEAW technique by Lim (2001). Studying 60 cases treated by the inventor of the technique, the late Dr. Young Kim of Massachusetts, Lim found that with anterior open bite closed by extrusion and tipping of the maxillary and mandibular incisors, and intrusion of the molars, there was less EARR in the maxillary incisors even though the root apices were displaced an average of 2 mm both horizontally and vertically. The mandibular incisors had greater EARR than the maxillary incisors. The study by Motokawa et al. (2013) furthermore showed that increased EARR in MEAW cases was also related to increased treatment time and increased time in elastics and amount of apical displacement.

Clinical Case 3 Anterior Open Bite
14-year-old female. CC: "fix my front teeth." High school student. Seasonal rhinitis. No history of trauma. No syndromes. First in family to have orthodontia. Skeletal dental Class II (ANB = 4.4°, molars quarter step Class II) with maxillary excess.

Maxillary incisors proclined by all measures including Steiner, Tweed, etc., with lip strain. Anterior open bite (see model). Forward tongue posture. "My front teeth have never touched." Good oral hygiene. No Bolton tooth size discrepancy. Maxillary central incisors are rotated mesially. PAN: all teeth present, third molars developing. Maxillary central incisor roots are <u>short</u> and pointed or bottle shaped. Initial records (Figs. 9, 10, and 11).

Narrative:

The treatment plan that was carried out included the extraction of first bicuspids to address crowding and incisor position. Patient and parents received extensive counseling by a myofunctional therapist to correct tongue posture. The training was marginally successful. A tongue "crib" was also used. The appliance was a 0.022 SWA. A palatal bar was placed but no headgear for vertical control. Total treatment time was 32 months. Patient wore elastics for finishing—anterior box and W for approximately 3 months. Case finished to ABO standards (Figs. 12, 13, and 14).

Note several interesting features of this case. EARR of 2–3 mm is noted on the maxillary central incisors and all four second bicuspids (Fig. 14). A rounding of the pointed ends of most of the teeth can be seen. Maxillary incisors were mostly tipped palatally with minimal displacement of the apices; however, the teeth were also rotated 30°.

Progress X-rays were not taken. The amount of EARR is moderate even though the crown root ratio of the central incisors is probably less than one. There was no mobility 3 months after treatment was completed. An interesting secondary finding was the increased room from mesial molar movement increasing the chance that the mandibular third molars will erupt normally.

Fig. 9 Initial cephalometric tracing

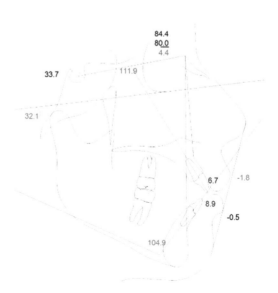

Fig. 10 Initial
study models

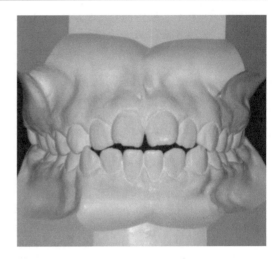

Fig. 11 Initial panoramic
radiograph

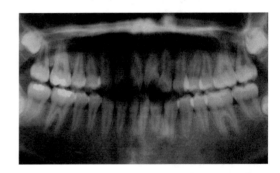

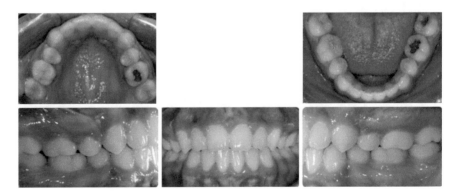

Fig. 12 Final extraoral images

Fig. 13 Final
cephalometric tracing

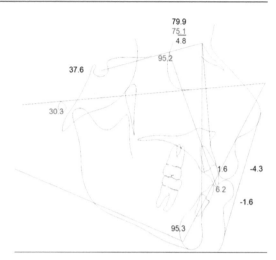

Fig. 14 Final panoramic
radiograph

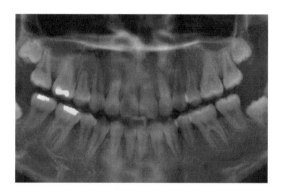

Were there any biomechanics that affected the EARR? A straight wire appliance was used and the largest archwires were TMA 0.019 × 0.025. Space closure was done on round wires. Finishing wires were steel round wires with elastics as noted previously.

2.5   Excess Overjet

The risk of developing EARR was found to be higher in patients with increased overjet in the majority of studies—this is probably a cofactor with extractions and apical displacement (Sameshima and Sinclair 2001a, b; Brin et al. 2003).

2.6   Patient Characteristics

1. Age: The literature is ambivalent, but most studies show no significant difference in age assuming that tooth formation including apex closure is mature and
   complete (e.g., Sameshima and Sinclair 2001a, b). Han et al. (2019) found no
   difference in EARR comparing "middle-aged" adults and young adults.
   Biologically there is trend toward increasing thickness of cementum; however
   root do not "grow" longer as we age.
2. Gender: it was once thought that females had a higher risk in males, but the literature overwhelmingly finds no significant differences in gender.
3. Ethnicity: through the discipline of dental anthropology, it is known that tooth
   and root variation is present among ethnically diverse populations. See Table 2
   EARR and ethnicity. Only one study has studied ethnicity as a risk factor for
   EARR (Sameshima and Sinclair 2002) who found that "Hispanic" patients had
   more EARR than Caucasians or Asians. A recent study by Wang et al. (2019)
   investigated crown to root ratios retrospectively in 333 patients. They found that
   "Hispanic" patients had significantly greater crown to root ratios than Caucasian
   or African American subjects did. The thesis by Nayak (2018) also found that
   Hispanic patients had a higher frequency of short root anomaly. Kennedy (2006)
   and Rojas (2008) found that subjects of Central American ancestry and subjects
   in Mexico City had much earlier eruption of the permanent dentition compared to
   non-Hispanic groups. Could the protective effect of the immature apex be lost
   earlier? This speculation in combination with shorter roots indicates that Hispanic
   patients are at relatively higher risk than other ethnicities, at least in North
   America.

Clinical Case 4

The patient was a 61-year-old adult Caucasian male in reasonably good health with
a history of regular dental examination and care. He had never had any orthodontic
treatment, but he paid for his three children to have orthodontia when they were
teens. His chief complaint was "I always wanted to have braces." The patient presented with a skeletal Class II malocclusion with 6 mm of crowding in the anterior
mandibular segment. Canine and molar relationships were Class I. All 32 teeth are
present on the initial examination. Risk factors for EARR would include dilacerated
roots for the maxillary incisors (Figs. 15 and 16).

Table 2 EARR and ethnicity

	Caucasians (mm)	Asians (mm)	Hispanics (mm)
Max. central incisors	1.32	0.78	1.64
Max. lateral incisors	1.65	1.02	1.69
Max. canines	1.11	0.84	1.59
Mand. central incisors	0.65	0.63	0.86
Mand. lateral incisors	0.81	0.67	1.08
Mand. canines	0.88	0.93	1.06

Fig. 15 Initial PAN

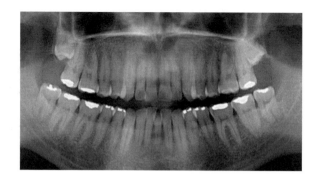

Fig. 16 Initial
cephalometric tracing

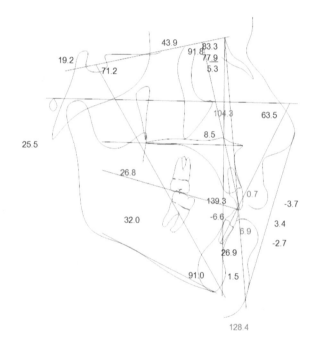

To resolve crowding a mandibular central incisor was extracted. An 0.022 SWA self-ligating bracket appliance was bonded from 6 to 6. Patient hygiene and cooperation were excellent. Treatment time was 18 months. The teeth appeared to move more slowly than normal, and the patient admitted taking OTC anti-inflammatory medications daily. The maxillary incisors were flared slightly, and ideal overbite and overjet were achieved. There was 3–4 mm of EARR on all three remaining mandibular incisors. Figure 17 apical root displacement was estimated to be 1–2 mm in the mesial distal direction. There is also a small but visible amount of EARR on the maxillary left central and lateral incisor.

The case is shown as a reminder that patients at any age may get significant EARR.

Fig. 17 Final PAN

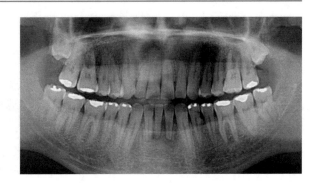

2.7   History of Trauma

Historically one of the first "risk factors" to the extent that clinicians would avoid moving teeth orthodontically that had such a positive history. It was also thought that teeth with a blunted apex had already had EARR due to trauma. It is now known that the evidence does not support this premise. Brin et al. (2003) reported that *there was no difference in the incidence of EARR between teeth that had had trauma and those that had not.*

3   Treatment Risk Factors

3.1   Apical Displacement

Clinical Case 5 Apical Displacement in a Non-extraction Case
The 24-year-old female patient presented with a Class I malocclusion with the chief complaint of crooked teeth. Here is a straightforward case with no apparent risk factors (Fig. 18). Non-extraction treatment with a 0.018 SWA appliance and the usual sequence of archwires was planned and completed in 18 months, finishing in ideal stainless steel archwires in order to achieve ideal torque and tip. The apex was estimated to have been intruded 1 mm and horizontally displaced 0.5 mm forward. The maxillary incisor EARR was 2–3 mm (Fig. 19). This case is a good example of apical displacement from palatal root torque associated with EARR.

Clinical Case 6
This case illustrates the finding that even with minor tooth movement and no risk factors, there are patients who fall under the "unexplained" category. The 32-year-old Asian male presented with a Class I malocclusion and chief complaint of "I do not like my front teeth." Figure 20, non-extraction treatment of normal treatment duration, resulted in generalized mild EARR—radiographically seen in Fig. 21 as a rounding of the more pointed root apices seen pretreatment.

From our understanding of the biology and physiology of tooth movement, apical displacement would seem to be the most logical major risk factor. Almost every

Fig. 18 Initial panoramic radiograph (Clinical Case 5)

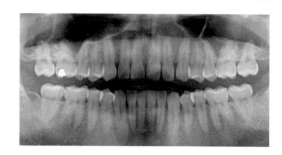

Fig. 19 Final panoramic radiograph (Clinical Case 5)

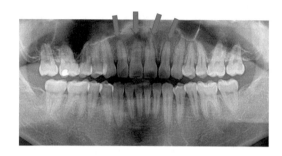

Fig. 20 Initial panoramic radiograph (Clinical Case 6)

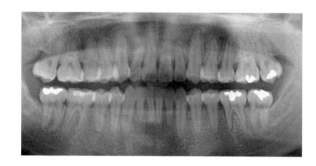

Fig. 21 Final panoramic radiograph (Clinical Case 6)

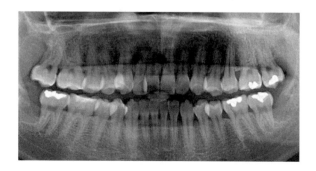

study that has included this measurement has concluded that duration of treatment is highly associated with EARR (Baumrind et al. 1996; Sameshima and Sinclair 2001a, b; van Loenen et al. 2007; Kim et al. 2018). In fact, there are many published studies claiming to have found EARR risk factors that completely ignore apical displacement; the findings of these papers must be considered weak at best. Measuring apical displacement was historically accomplished by superimposing cephs. This is fraught with inaccuracy, but if done carefully and checked quantitatively using established statistical methods, superimposition can yield useful results. More recently, investigators have been trying to use 3D volumes to achieve the same purpose, but the methods have proven to be neither precise nor accurate (see chapter "Imaging of External Apical Root Resorption"). A recent study examining mesially moved first molars showed that EARR occurs with significant distances (Winkler et al. 2017).

Clinical Case 7 Apical Displacement
The patient was treated with fixed appliances for 25 months for a Class I malocclusion. Four bicuspids were extracted for crowding and protrusive teeth and lip strain. Roots were long and narrow with dilacerations present in many teeth; however, no other risk factors were present. Figure 22 illustrated the manner in which apical displacement may be calculated on superimposed pre- and post-treatment tracings. A comparison between pre- and post-treatment periapical radiographs of the anterior teeth showed >4 mm EARR on both maxillary central incisors (Figs. 23 and 24).

Maxillary incisor root contacting palatal bone: widely reported was a study that showed that moving the roots of the maxillary incisors to the endosteal surface of the palatal cortical bone was a significant factor in EARR (Kaley and Phillips 1991). Subsequent investigations have neither confirmed nor denied the association (Mirabella and Artun 1995), and it is probable that it is a secondary finding to apical displacement (true distance moved).

Maxillary central incisor roots contacting the incisive or nasopalatine canal. Cho et al. (2016) found that the apex of the central incisor was on average 5–6 mm distance from the canal. In a study of untreated subjects using CBCT images, Matsumura et al. (2017) found that the apex of the maxillary incisor on average was 4 mm away from the incisive canal. This is a distance that is rarely achieved in apical displacement horizontally. Two case reports from Chung et al. (2015) found EARR for one of the central incisors that had made direct contact with the cortical plate of the incisive canal; the amount of apical displacement was facilitated with the use of orthodontic mini-implants.

3.2   Prolonged Treatment Time

Treatment time or treatment duration has long been suspected of being a risk factor for EARR. In chapter "Etiology" the basis of this factor was described scientifically through the work of Al-Qawasmi et al. (2003), in which patients with inborn vulnerability have a lower threshold of remodeling cycles before the system of protection

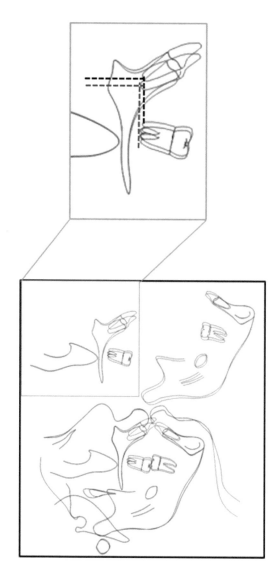

Fig. 22 Superimposition of pre- and post-treatment tracings to calculate the amount of apical displacement. In this case the maxillary central incisor root apex was displaced 1.6 mm distally and intruded 1.4 mm

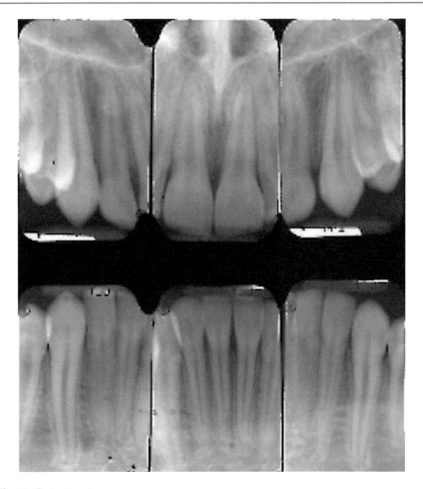

Fig. 23 Pretreatment

from EARR breaks down. The majority of EARR studies that have included this variable found an association between treatment duration and EARR (Sameshima and Sinclair 2001a, b, 2004; Vlaskalic et al. 1998; Brezniak and Wasserstein 2002; Kaley and Phillips 1991; Pandis et al. 2008).

Clinical Case 8 Prolonged Treatment Duration (Fig. 25)
This patient was a 34-year-old female at the start of treatment. CC: mild maxillary crowding and rotations and impacted mandibular left second premolar. The orthodontist elected to bring in the impacted tooth despite the patient's age (pretreatment records were not available, and transfer radiographs were "lost"). Patient transferred when the orthodontist retired 3 years in. There was sufficient space, but the pathway was incorrect, and insufficient bone was removed by the periodontist who did the closed exposure. The crown of the premolar damaged the root of the first molar. The

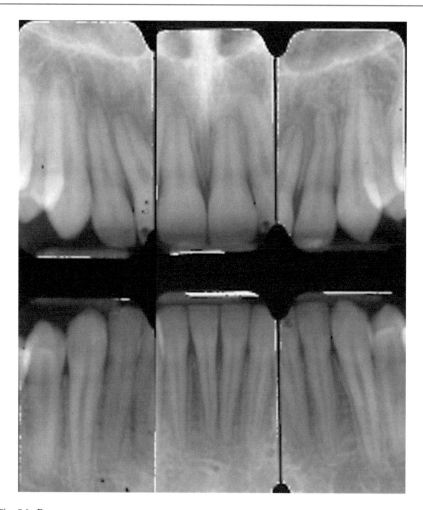

Fig. 24 Post-treatment

Fig. 25 Final PAN and (inset) progress periapical at transfer (Clinical Case 8)

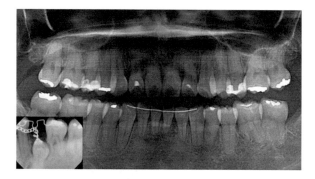

second orthodontist replaced the appliance and 2 years later finished the case. Note generalized root resorption and moderate to severe EARR for the maxillary and mandibular incisors. The classic paper by Becker and Chaushu (2003) strongly suggested that moving impacted teeth in patients over the age of 30 is ill-advised and futile.

3.3   Extraction Cases

If extractions are done for any reason, this has been found to be a risk factor for EARR (Sameshima and Sinclair 2001a, b). The risk does not appear to vary among extraction patterns, i.e., if you extract first bicuspids, second bicuspids, or upper bicuspids only (Sameshima and Sinclair 2001a, b), there is no distinction. Statistically it is less certain if the extraction factor is independent of other factors such as apical displacement. In maxillary bicuspid extractions only for Class II cases with excess overjet, the distance the apex moves is the dominant consideration.

Clinical Case 9 Extraction Case
Class I skeletal mild crowding with chief complaint of "I don't like my smile." This is a 15.5-year-old female with a negative health history. The maxillary incisor root shapes are slightly pointed, and there is a small dilaceration at the apex of the maxillary right lateral incisor (Fig. 26). Four first bicuspids were extracted. Ideal torque was achieved in the maxillary anterior segment. Ideal overjet and overbite were accomplished. Note approximately 3 mm EARR for all four maxillary incisors. They were displaced approximately 2.2 mm horizontally (Fig. 27).

Case 10 Extraction Case
The patient was a healthy 18.1-year-old Caucasian female with a skeletal Class III malocclusion. Problem list included mild crowding in both arches, flared maxillary incisors, Class III molar relationship, misaligned and rotated teeth, and impacted third molars (Fig. 28). Treatment plan: extract maxillary second bicuspids, mandibular first bicuspids, and bond a 0.022 staight-wire appliance.

Fig. 26 Initial panoramic radiograph (Clinical Case 9)

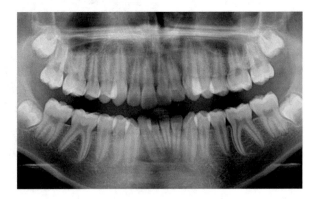

Maxillary first and mandibular second bicuspids were extracted to facilitate Class I relations. Finishing elastics and steel final archwires. Note rounding of the apices of the maxillary incisors (<2 mm EARR) (Fig. 29). Thirty months total treatment time. 1 mm horizontal and vertical apical displacement—see Fig. 30 superimposed tracings.

Case 11 Extraction Case

15-year-old male. CC: "crooked front teeth stick out." Health history negative. No history of trauma. Class II Div 1 malocclusion with deep bite and excess overjet.

Fig. 27 Final panoramic radiograph (Clinical Case 9)

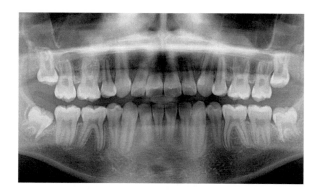

Fig. 28 Initial PAN (Clinical Case 10 Extraction Case)

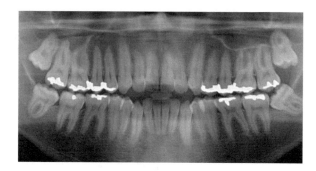

Fig. 29 Final PAN (Clinical Case 10 Extraction Case)

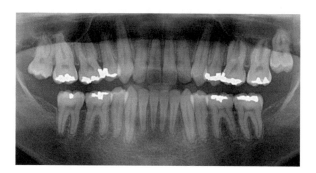

Fig. 30 Superimposition
to show 2 mm intrusion
and 2 mm posterior
horizontal displacement of
the maxillary central
incisor apex

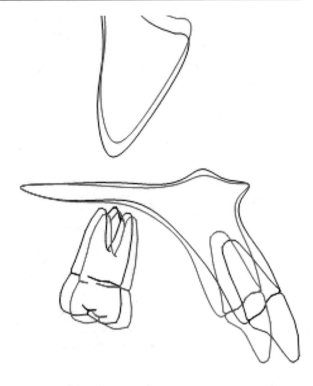

Fig. 31 Initial PAN
(Clinical Case 11)

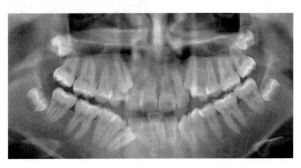

Full step Class II molars. Severe crowding in both arches with blocked out canines. Note pointed and dilacerated roots on all four maxillary incisors. In this initial PAN, the mandibular incisor roots are distorted and look short (Figs. 31 and 32).

Moderate to severe EARR on all four maxillary incisors is apparent. Total treatment time was 33 months. Appliance was MBT 0.022. Ideal incisor position (torque) as a goal was achieved. Was extraction a factor by itself?

3.4 Absolute Intrusion with Skeletal Anchorage

Teeth can be intruded or moved previously unheard of distances using skeletal anchorage. For molar intrusion to close anterior open bite, there is some evidence that EARR can occur similar to the way apical displacement is a factor for other teeth. The thesis by Kim (2018) showed EARR on nearly every molar studied using CBCT material in molar intrusion for open bite (Figs. 33, 34, and 35). Similar findings were shown in work by Liou and Chang (2010) and Heravi et al. (2011). What happens to the apex when the tooth is intruded into the sinus? This question is not well studied, but an interesting animal study was done in Japan by Daimaruya et al. (2003) in which they intruded teeth in dogs 4 mm. The root apex penetrated the nasal floor; there was "moderate" EARR and interestingly, they found that new bone formed over the intruded root.

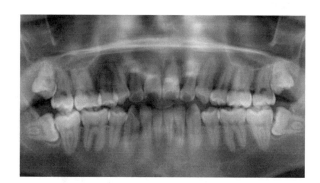

Fig. 32 Final PAN (Clinical Case 11)

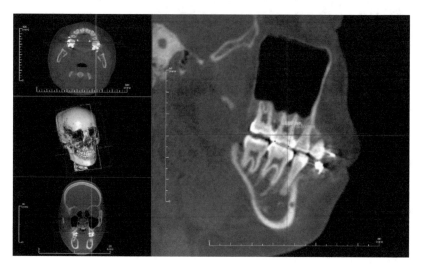

Fig. 33 Pretreatment molar intrusion (Clinical Case 12)

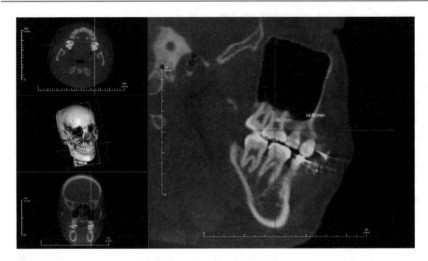

Fig. 34 Post-treatment molar intrusion case—CBCT slice through the buccal roots of the maxillary first molar

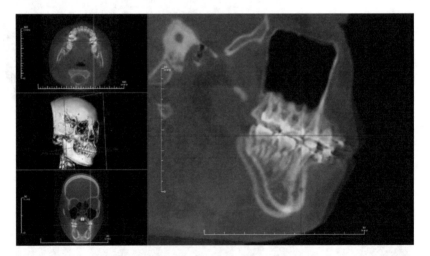

Fig. 35 Superimposed volumes on best fit coronal structures. Note auto rotation of mandible

Clinical Case 12 Molar Intrusion with Skeletal Anchorage Devices

The patient presented with a skeletal anterior open bite (Fig. 33). Careful diagnosis showed that by intruding the maxillary posterior teeth, bite closure could be achieved without compromising the airway, thus avoiding two jaw surgery. Figure 34 shows the final CBCT with successful treatment of the anterior open bite as planned. Figure 35 shows the pre- and post-treatment volumes superimposed on a "best fit of stable structures" method.

Change in root length: Mesial buccal root = −0.7 mm

Distal buccal root = −1.3 mm

It also appears that remodeling of bone and periosteum has occurred over the root apices in the floor of the sinus.

Clinical Case 13 Absolute Intrusion of Posterior Teeth Using Plate Anchorage
This adult patient also presented with a skeletal anterior open bite. VTOs suggested intrusion with skeletal anchorage would have a high degree of success in closing the bite non-surgically. The patient agreed to the placement of zygomatic plates. 32 months of treatment were required to close the anterior open bite. The roots of the teeth were long with some dilacerations at the beginning of treatment (Fig. 36). There were no changes at progress (Fig. 37). At the end of treatment, the maxillary molars were intruded approximately 2–3 mm (Fig. 38). There is a moderate degree of EARR on all four maxillary molars (<2.5 mm). There is also a generalized rounding of the apex in all teeth.

3.5   Heavy Forces

Clinically it would make sense that so-called light forces would produce less EARR, but the question is more complicated than it seems (Ren et al. 2003). Firstly, it is

Fig. 36 Pretreatment PAN (Clinical Case 13)

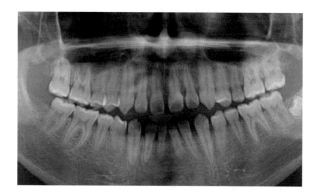

Fig. 37 Progress PAN—after leveling and aligning (Clinical Case 13)

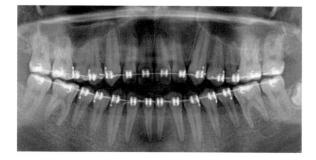

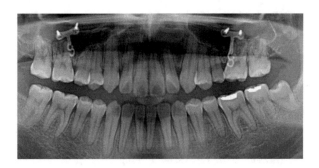

Fig. 38 Post-treatment PAN (Clinical Case 13)

difficult to quantify forces placed on the root. Second, individual response to forces is highly variable, i.e., the same force applied to a tooth may result in resorption in one person but not the next person. And third, and most important, as stated in chapter "Etiology", the root apex is different from the root surface. Veteran clinicians who have seen methods evolve from the standard appliance all steel archwire era to the straight-wire novel metals era have probably observed a great reduction in EARR in their cases. Certainly the heavy torque and heavy forces produced by closing loops and the additional forces applied from elastics and anchorage methods would stress the system to capacity.

3.6   Interoffice Differences

Only one study looked at interoffice differences in EARR prevalence, and it was determined that there is significant differences after statistically accounting for individual office variation in known risk factors. Unfortunately, some offices for some as yet to be determined reason have more EARR than others (Sameshima and Sinclair 2001a, b).

3.7   Selected Topics

3.7.1   Clear Aligners

The small amount of tooth movement induced at each stage of clear aligner therapy seemed promising as far as lessening the amount of EARR. However, with the advances in aligner mechanics, it is now apparent that if there is root apex displacement, then the amount of EARR will be no different from that with fixed appliances (Iglesias-Linares et al. 2017; Gay et al. 2017).

A thesis by Fowler (2010) showed no EARR with clear aligners, but in none of the clear aligner cases was there any apical displacement. Two studies claiming to show less EARR with clear aligners (Aman et al. 2018; Eissa et al. 2018; Li et al. 2020) did not report apical displacement, a common problem with most studies. A randomized clinical trial with clear aligners found the effect on cementum was similar when compared to fixed treatment (Barbagallo et al 2008).

3.7.2 Accelerated Tooth Movement

In 2020, there are several claimed methods for accelerating tooth movement. The evidence is poor either way for risk for EARR. Theoretically, if the inflammatory process necessary for accelerating bone turnover/wound healing is increased, it would be reasonable to conclude that the same processes would be at work at the root apex.

3.7.3 New Bracket Systems

There is no longer any question that self-ligation systems do not produce less EARR. The number of studies that have refuted the claim is compelling, e.g., Pandis et al. (2008), Handem et al. (2016), Jacobs et al. (2014), and Chen et al. (2015). Any bracket system or device that claims to reduce EARR must show evidence in the form of controlled well-design clinical experiments and moreover present a strong scientific foundation verified by expert, neutral evaluation.

No difference was found in labial vs lingual appliances (Nassif et al. 2017; Pamukçu et al. 2020). An interesting finding was more EARR was found in the mandibular teeth in lingual cases (Pamukçu et al. 2020).

4 Suspected Risk Factors

4.1 Maxillofacial Surgery Cases

There have been a number of testimonials regarding the prevalence of EARR in orthognathic surgery cases, in particular, Le Fort I surgery and its effect on the maxillary incisors. The biological basis was compromised blood supply and a rapid regional bone turnover similar to what is seen in a certain type of accelerated tooth movement. But also maxillary incisors usually have to be detorqued in order to decompensate the malocclusion, and this would increase risk due to apical displacement. Mirabella and Artun (1995) found no association for EARR with maxillary surgery. A study comparing surgery vs non-surgery patients specifically found that EARR was significantly higher in the surgery group for maxillary lateral incisors (Watson 2006). The same paper reported that there was no relationship between EARR and "specific type of surgery including interdental osteotomies, use or duration of a surgical splint, type or duration of MMF, or the particular dentofacial deformity being treated."

Clinical Case 14
This interesting case documents the orthodontic treatment of a patient for 16 years. EARR occurred during fixed orthodontic therapy, while the patient was a teen. Despite a number of interventions, the main feature and complaint of anterior open bite resisted resolution until finally she had orthognathic surgery as an adult.

The patient was a 10.5-year-old Caucasian female who presented with chief complaint of open bite. Clinically she presented with Class I mixed dentition malocclusion featuring high, blocked out maxillary canines and an anterior open bite from canines (see initial PAN and periapicals—Fig. 39). Phase I treatment—myofunctional therapy and tongue crib—was planned and carried out. Her health history was negative, and there was no family history of orthognathic surgery.

In Fig. 40 the patient was ready to start Phase II. The anterior open bite was unresolved. The roots of the permanent maxillary incisors are thin, and the right central incisor apex is indistinct. The apex of the left central incisor is mildly pointed.

After 2 years of Phase II treatment consisting of fixed appliances and many weeks of wearing elastics including up and downs with limited success treatment was stopped. See Fig. 41. EARR is noted particularly severe on all four maxillary incisors.

Six years after the previous records were taken, the patient is 23 years old. See Fig. 42. She has a posterior crossbite and anterior open bite. There is no further EARR. The decision was made to set up the case for orthognathic surgery.

In Fig. 43, after the successful completion of orthodontic and orthognathic surgery (two jaw), the patient is 26. Prognosis of these teeth? See chapter 9 "Long Term Prognosis".

Though not documented well, there is often significant EARR of the maxillary incisors in Le Fort I maxillary surgery cases, but in this case the EARR occurred many years prior to surgery. Chapter 6 "Imaging of External Apical Root Resorption", Figs. 12, 13, 14, 15, 16, 17, 18, 19, and 20, illustrates severe EARR with surgically assisted rapid maxillary expansion.

Fig. 39 Initial panoramic and periapical radiographs (Clinical Case 14)

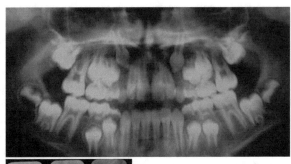

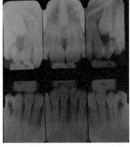

Fig. 40 Progress PAN and periapicals taken 2 years later

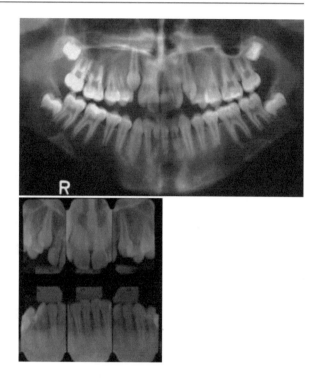

Fig. 41 Final panoramic and periapical radiographs at the conclusion of Phase II (Clinical Case 14)

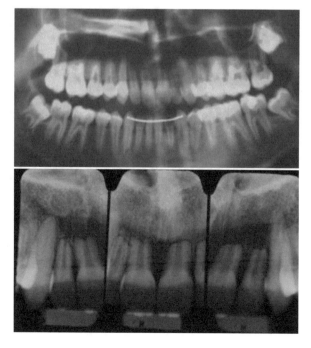

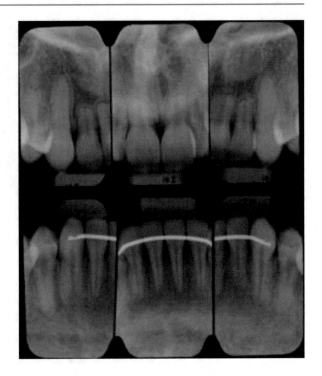

Fig. 42 These periapicals (above) were taken at age 23

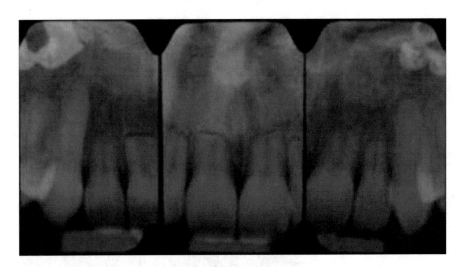

Fig. 43 Final (post-surgery) periapical radiographs (Clinical Case 14)

5   Factors Not Considered Increased Risk

A number of mechanical factors that were thought to be risk factors have been studied and found not to be significant. These include treatment philosophy, bracket type, slot size, headgear, functional appliances, malocclusion type, archwire type or sequence, etc. Apical displacement and treatment duration ultimately account for the greatest risk, and these mechanical factors are secondary or tertiary.

Two treatment factors that have not been well studied but may be less riskier for EARR than originally thought are any form of rapid maxillary expansion and use of intermaxillary elastics. Akyalcin et al. (2015), using CBCT data, found that RME does not increase the risk of EARR. The systematic review of expansion and EARR by Forst et al. (2014) found no significant difference from three papers that qualified for the review. The risk of EARR is of far less concern than causing a fenestration or dehiscence. Wear of intermaxillary elastics, especially for vertical control, has long been felt to be a significant factor in orthodontics over the many years; however, the displacement of the apex in these cases is most likely the main cause and would explain what clinicians used to call "jiggling," i.e., sporadic wear of elastics during finishing stages.

References

Akyalcin S, Alexander SP, Silva RM, English JD. Evaluation of three-dimensional root surface changes and resorption following rapid maxillary expansion: a cone beam computed tomography investigation. Orthod Craniofac Res. 2015;18(Suppl 1):117–26.

Al-Qawasmi RA, Hartsfield JK Jr, Everett ET, Flury L, Liu L, Foroud TM, Macri JV, Roberts WE. Genetic predisposition to external apical root resorption. Am J Orthod Dentofac Orthop. 2003;123(3):242–52.

Aman C, Azevedo B, Bednar E, Chandiramami S, German D, Nicholson E, Ni-cholson K, Scarfe WC. Apical root resorption during orthodontic treatment with clear aligners: a retrospective study using cone-beam computed tomography. Am J Orthod Dentofac Orthop. 2018;153(6):842–51.

Barbagallo LJ, Jones AS, Petocz P, Darendeliler MA. Physical properties of root cementum: part 10. Comparison of the effects of invisible removable thermoplastic appliances with light and heavy orthodontic forces on premolar cementum. A microcomputed-tomography study. Am J Orthod Dentofac Orthop. 2008;133(2):218–27.

Baumrind S, Korn EL, Boyd RL. Apical root resorption in orthodontically treated adults. Am J Orthod Dentofac Orthop. 1996;110(3):311–20. https://doi.org/10.1016/s0889-5406(96)80016-3.

Becker A, Chaushu S. Success rate and duration of orthodontic treatment for adult patients with palatally impacted maxillary canines. Am J Orthod Dentofac Orthop. 2003;124(5):509–14.

Brezniak N, Wasserstein A. Orthodontically induced inflammatory root resorption. Part II: the clinical aspects. Angle Orthod. 2002;72(2):180–4. Review

Brin I, Ben-Bassat Y, Heling I, Engelberg A. The influence of orthodontic treatment on previously traumatized permanent incisors. Eur J Orthod. 1991;13(5):372–7.

Brin I, Tulloch JF, Koroluk L, Philips C. External apical root resorption in Class II malocclusion: a retrospective review of 1- versus 2-phase treatment. Am J Orthod Dentofacial Orthop. 2003;124(2):151–6.

Chen W, Haq AA, Zhou Y. Root resorption of self-ligating and conventional preadjusted brackets in severe anterior crowding Class I patients: a longitudinal retrospective study. BMC Oral Health. 2015;15:115.

Cho EA, Kim SJ, Choi YJ, Kim KH, Chung CJ. Morphologic evaluation of the incisive canal and its proximity to the maxillary central incisors using computed tomography images. Angle Orthod. 2016;86(4):571–6.

Chung CJ, Choi YJ, Kim KH. Approximation and contact of the maxillary central incisor roots with the incisive canal after maximum retraction with temporary anchorage devices: Report of 2 patients. Am J Orthod Dentofac Orthop. 2015;148(3):493–502.

Daimaruya T, Takahashi I, Nagasaka H, Umemori M, Sugawara J, Mitani H. Effects of maxillary molar intrusion on the nasal floor and tooth root using the skeletal anchorage system in dogs. Angle Orthod. 2003;73(2):158–66.

Davidovitch Z, Lee YJ, Counts AL, Park YG, Bursac Z. The immune system possibly modulates orthodontic root resorption. In: Davidovitch Z, Mah J, editors. Biological mechanisms of tooth movement and craniofacial adaptation. Boston: Harvard Society for the Advancement of Orthodontics; 2000. p. 207–17.

Edward F. Harris, Monte L. Butler. Patterns of incisor root resorption before and after orthodontic correction in cases with anterior open bites. American Journal of Orthodontics and Dentofacial Orthopedics. 1992;101(2):112–119.

Eissa O, Carlyle T, El-Bialy T. Evaluation of root length following treatment with clear aligners and two different fixed orthodontic appliances. A pilot study. J Orthod Sci. 2018;7:11.

Fernandes LQP, Figueiredo NC, Montalvany Antonucci CC, Lages EMB, Andrade I Jr, Capelli Junior J. Predisposing factors for external apical root resorption associated with orthodontic treatment. Korean J Orthod. 2019;49(5):310–8.

Forst D, Nijjar S, Khaled Y, Lagravere M, Flores-Mir C. Radiographic assessment of external root resorption associated with jackscrew-based maxillary expansion therapies: a systematic review. Eur J Orthod. 2014;36(5):576–85.

Fowler B. A comparison of root resorption between invisalign treatment and contemporary orthodontic treatment. [Thesis]. University of Southern California. 2010.

Gay G, Ravera S, Castroflorio T, Garino F, Rossini G, Parrini S, Cugliari G, Deregibus A. Root resorption during orthodontic treatment with Invisalign®: a radiometric study. Prog Orthod. 2017;18(1):12.

Han J, Hwang S, Nguyen T, Proffit WR, Soma K, Choi YJ, Kim KH, Chung CJ. Periodontal and root changes after orthodontic treatment in middle-aged adults are similar to those in young adults. Am J Orthod Dentofac Orthop. 2019;155(5):650–5.

Handem RH, Janson G, Matias M, de Freitas KM, de Lima DV, Garib DG, de Freitas MR. External root resorption with the self-ligating Damon system—a retrospective study. Prog Orthod. 2016;17(1):20.

Heravi F, Bayani S, Madani AS, Radvar M, Anbiaee N. Intrusion of supra-erupted molars using miniscrews: clinical success and root resorption. Am J Orthod Dentofac Orthop. 2011;139(4 Suppl):S170–5.

Iglesias-Linares A, Sonnenberg B, Solano B, Yañez-Vico RM, Solano E, Lindauer SJ, Flores-Mir C. Orthodontically induced external apical root resorption in patients treated with fixed appliances vs removable aligners. Angle Orthod. 2017;87(1):3–10.

Jacobs C, Gebhardt PF, Jacobs V, Hechtner M, Meila D, Wehrbein H. Root resorption, treatment time and extraction rate during orthodontic treatment with self-ligating and conventional brackets. Head Face Med. 2014;10:2.

Kaley J, Phillips C. Factors related to root resorption in edgewise practice. Angle Orthod. 1991;61:125–32.

Kamble RH, Lohkare S, Hararey PV, Mundada RD. Stress distribution pattern in a root of maxillary central incisor having various root morphologies: a finite element study. Angle Orthod. 2012;82(5):799–805.

Kennedy DM. Early eruption of the permanent dentition in Hispanic adolescents [thesis]. University of Southern California, Los Angeles. 2006.

Kim J, Sameshima GT. Three-dimensional assessment of EARR associated with molar intrusion. [Thesis]. University of Southern California. 2018.

Kim KW, Kim SJ, Lee JY, Choi YJ, Chung CJ, Lim H, Kim KH. Apical root displacement is a critical risk factor for apical root resorption after orthodontic treatment. Angle Orthod. 2018;88:740–7.

Kindelan SA, Day PF, Kindelan JD, Spencer JR, Duggal MS. Dental trauma: an overview of its influence on the management of orthodontic treatment. Part 1. J Orthod. 2008;35(2):68–78.

Kook YA, Park S, Sameshima GT. Peg-shaped and small lateral incisors not at higher risk for root resorption. Am J Orthod Dentofac Orthop. 2003;123(3):253–8.

Li Y, Deng S, Mei L, Li Z, Zhang X, Yang C, Li Y. Prevalence and severity of apical root resorption during orthodontic treatment with clear aligners and fixed appliances: a cone beam computed tomography study. Prog Orthod. 2020;21(1):1.

Lim R. Evaluation of root resorption after the multiloop edgewise archwire (MEAW) appliance in patients with anterior open bites [thesis]. University of Southern California, Los Angeles. 2001.

Liou EJ, Chang PM. Apical root resorption in orthodontic patients with en-masse maxillary anterior retraction and intrusion with miniscrews. Am J Orthod Dentofac Orthop. 2010;137(2):207–12.

Matsumura T, Ishida Y, Kawabe A, Ono T. Quantitative analysis of the relationship between maxillary incisors and the incisive canal by cone-beam computed tomography in an adult Japanese population. Prog Orthod. 2017;18(1):24.

McNab S, Battistutta D, Taverne A, Symons AL. External apical root resorption of posterior teeth in asthmatics after orthodontic treatment. Am J Orthod Dentofac Orthop. 1999;116(5):545–51.

Mirabella AD, Artun J. Risk factors for apical root resorption of maxillary anterior teeth in adult orthodontic patients. Am J Orthod Dentofacial Orthop. 1995;108(1):48–55.

Mitchell CA, Kennedy JG, Wallace RG. Dental abnormalities associated with familial expansile osteolysis: a clinical and radiographic study. Oral Surg Oral Med Oral Pathol. 1990;70(3):301–7.

Motokawa M, Terao A, Kaku M, Kawata T, Gonzales C, Darendeliler MA, Tanne K. Open bite as a risk factor for orthodontic root resorption. Eur J Orthod. 2013;35:790–5.

Murata N, Ioi H, Ouchi M, Takao T, Oida H, Aijima R, Yamaza T, Kido MA. Effect of allergen sensitization on external root resorption. J Dent Res. 2013;92(7):641–7.

Nassif CE, Cotrim-Ferreira A, Conti ACCF, Valarelli DP, de Almeida Cardoso M, de Almeida-Pedrin RR. Comparative study of root resorption of maxillary incisors in patients treated with lingual and buccal orthodontics. Angle Orthod. 2017;87(6):795–800.

Nayak SC. Interleukin-1 beta (il-1β) gene polymorphisms in pre-treatment orthodontic patients exhibiting short root anomaly (SRA) [thesis]. University of Las Vegas Nevada, Las Vegas. 2018.

Nishioka M, Ioi H, Nakata S, Nakasima A, Counts A. Root resorption and immune system factors in the Japanese. Angle Orthod. 2006;76(1):103–8.

Owman-Moll P, Kurol J. Root resorption after orthodontic treatment in high-and low-risk patients: analysis of allergy as a possible predisposing factor. Eur J Orthod. 2000;22(6):657–63.

Pamukçu H, Polat-Özsoy Ö, Gülşahi A, Özemre MÖ. External apical root resorption after non-extraction orthodontic treatment with labial vs. lingual fixed appliances. J Orofac Orthop. 2020;81(1):41–51.

Pandis N, Nasika M, Polychronopoulou A, Eliades T. External apical root resorption in patients treated with conventional and self-ligating brackets. Am J Orthod Dentofac Orthop. 2008;134(5):646–51.

Ren Y, Maltha JC, Kuijpers-Jagtman AM. Optimum force magnitude for orthodontic tooth movement: a systematic literature review. Angle Orthod. 2003;73(1):86–92.

Rivera EM, Walton RE. Extensive idiopathic apical root resorption. A case report. Oral Surg Oral Med Oral Pathol. 1994;78(5):673–7.

Rojas J. Sexual differences and early eruption timing of the permanent dentition in Mexican adolescents—a comparison with Caucasian standards [thesis]. University of Southern California, Los Angeles. 2008.

Sameshima GT, Sinclair PM. Predicting and preventing root resorption: part I. Diagnostic factors. Am J Orthod Dentofac Orthop. 2001a;119(5):505–10.

Sameshima GT, Sinclair PM. Predicting and preventing root resorption: part II. Treatment factors. Am J Orthod Dentofac Orthop. 2001b;119(5):511–5.

Sameshima GT, Sinclair PM. Characteristics of patients with severe root resorption. Orthod Craniofac Res. 2004;7(2):108–14.

Shaw A, Sameshima GT, Vu H. Mechanical stress generated by orthodontic forces on apical root cementum: a finite element model. Orthod Craniofac Res. 2004;7(2):98–107.

van Loenen M, Dermaut LR, Degrieck J, De Pauw GA. Apical root resorption of upper incisors during the torquing stage of the tip-edge technique. Eur J Orthod. 2007;29(6):583–8.

Vlaskalic V, Boyd RL, Baumrind S. Etiology and sequelae of root resorption. Semin Orthod. 1998;4:124–31.

Wang J, Rousso C, Christensen BI, Li P, Kau CH, MacDougall M, Lamani E. Ethnic differences in the root to crown ratios of the permanent dentition. Orthod Craniofac Res. 2019;22(2):99–104.

Watson J. Apical root resorption of anterior teeth following orthognathic surgery. J Oral Maxillofacial Surg. 2006;64(9):52.

Winkler J, Göllner N, Göllner P, Pazera P, Gkantidis N. Apical root resorption due to mandibular first molar mesialization: a split-mouth study. Am J Orthod Dentofac Orthop. 2017;151(4):708–17.

Yu Zhou. Open bite as a risk factor for orthodontic root resorption. The European Journal of Orthodontics 2015;37(1):118.2–119.

Imaging of External Apical Root Resorption

Glenn T. Sameshima

1 Preface

EARR is essentially an asymptomatic condition; there is almost never pain or discomfort associated with short roots. There is clinically no distinction between tooth mobility and tooth length during orthodontic tooth movement. Therefore, radiographic images are necessary to diagnose and manage EARR.

2 2D Imaging of EARR

Periapical and panoramic radiographs have been used reliably for many years. The limitations are well documented, and there is a communal commonality in reading these films to determine EARR. Digital radiographs have greatly reduced exposure to ionizing radiation and made storage easier. There is no longer a need to process chemicals in the office, and the images can be enhanced greatly with proper software and a minimum of operator skill. The newer panoramic machines are user-friendly and greatly reduce the need for retakes. The advantages and disadvantages are summarized below:

Periapical Radiographs: Advantages
1. Widely available and universally interpretable
2. Relatively low cost
3. Relatively low radiation and environmentally friendly if digital
4. Can be adjusted with software for improved readability
5. Established methods for measuring root length

G. T. Sameshima (✉)
Advanced Orthodontics, Herman Ostrow School of Dentistry of the University of Southern California, Los Angeles, CA, USA
e-mail: sameshim@usc.edu

© Springer Nature Switzerland AG 2021
G. T. Sameshima (ed.), *Clinical Management of Orthodontic Root Resorption*,
https://doi.org/10.1007/978-3-030-58706-2_6

(a) Subjective
(b) Objective
6. Transportability and storage for digital images is good

Periapical Radiographs: Disadvantages
1. Two-dimensional image of three-dimensional structure
2. Variation in image quality
3. Cannot see some root dilaceration and irregularity in shape
4. Subject to distortion based on both method and systematic error

Panoramic Radiographs: Advantages
1. Also widely available
2. Easy to learn
3. Universal interpretation
4. Can see all the teeth in one view

Panoramic Films: Disadvantages
1. Machines can be costly.
2. Difficult to measure distances precisely.
3. Require calibration.
4. Difficult for some patients.

Most of the images used in this book are panoramic images. A standard set of initial orthodontic records in North America includes a panoramic film or FMXR and a lateral cephalometric film. For EARR panoramic films are generally acceptable assuming they are taken on a digital machine. Sameshima and Asgarifar (2003) found that root shape and measurement of EARR on pre- and post-treatment records of orthodontic patients were more accurate with periapical radiographs vs panoramic images. See Figs. 1, 2, and 3 which compares a PAN vs PAs. The panoramic images created from 3D volumes have improved but are still lacking in image quality and consistency when compared to standard digital panoramic images. To quantify EARR the best images are periapical radiographs taken by a skilled operator in a standardized fashion. On panoramic images, EARR must be measured using a nominal scale or estimated quantitatively by the clinician.

Fig. 1 Final panoramic film (original scanned under medium resolution using a flatbed scanner)

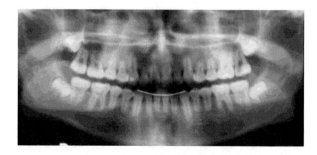

Fig. 2 Magnification of the panoramic film (unretouched) to show the maxillary incisor root apices

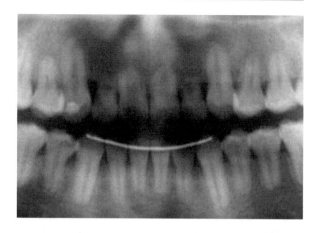

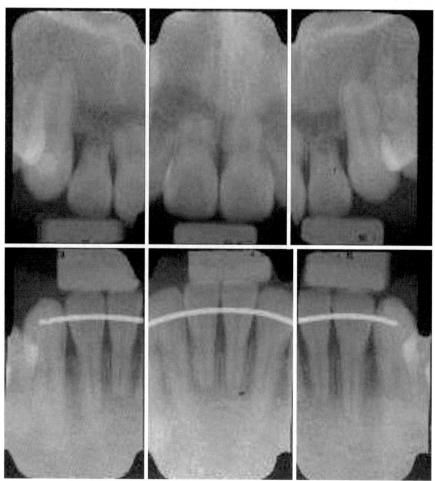

Fig. 3 Periapical films—originals scanned as in previous Fig. 1

3   Three-Dimensional Images

Cone beam CT scans (CBCT) have removed the problem of the periapical and panoramic two-dimensional representation of a 3D object (Fig. 4). The downside is the
quality of the image. There is a big "trade-off" between quality and amount of radiation exposure. The industry appears to have overcome the wild variation among
machines that bewildered clinicians when CBCT first arrived many years ago.
CBCT are commonly used now, and the software packages produce good diagnostic
images. Clinically it would seem obvious that 3D images would be superior to 2D
images for locating impacted teeth, but an influential study by Christell et al. (2018)
showed that clinicians' treatment decisions were the same regardless of whether
they looked at 2D images vs 3D images.

Figures 5, 6, and 7 is an old case but illustrates the advantages of visualization
teeth in three dimensions over two. Early studies by Sameshima and Sinclair (2004),

Fig. 4 Pre- and post-
treatment CBCT
comparison to illustrate the
diagnosis of severe EARR
using 3D images.
(Courtesy Dr. Jeong Ho
Choi, Seoul, Korea, and
Dr. James Mah, Las Vegas,
Nevada, USA)

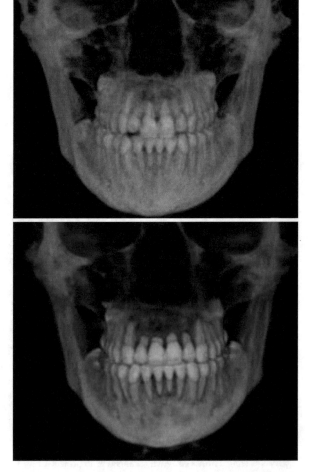

Fig. 5 Pretreatment PAN for orthodontics ("wet" film scanned for publication, hence the poor image quality)

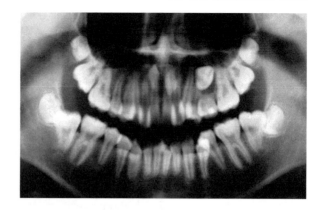

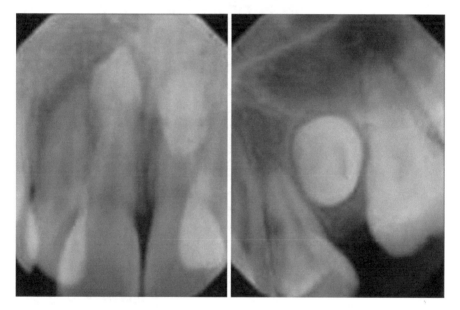

Fig. 6 Periapical radiographs taken by the restorative dentist. The dual mesiodens and the ectopic maxillary left second bicuspid are visible in both films, but their roots are not visible in either view. The resolution is superior in the periapical and bitewing x-rays. Note also the mandibular incisor distortion on the PAN: the roots appear shorter, and the small dilacerations cannot be seen

Nakajima et al. (2005), Walker et al. (2005), Peck et al. (2007), and others demonstrated the superiority of 3D images of roots over 2D images. Lund et al. (2010) showed that CBCT images had the advantage of providing the same information regardless of position of the scan. A paper authored by Kumar et al. (2011) compared the accuracy of identifying defects between periapical radiographs and CBCT images and found no significant differences. However, a thesis by Hecht (2013) showed conclusively that root dilaceration normal to the midsagittal plane is not detectable by 2D images but readily visualized on CBCT volumes. A systematic

Fig. 7 Two views from one CBCT volume. Soft tissue and some hard tissue have been removed virtually for maximal visualization of the dentition. Note the ectopic maxillary first bicuspid—the crown is palatal to the root, and the tooth is parallel to the occlusal plane

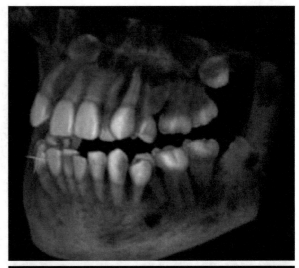

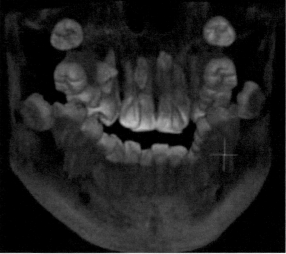

review of EARR studies that only employed CBCT found limited results not so different from systematic reviews with 2D study material (Samandara et al. 2019).

Figure 8 shows a pretreatment limited CBCT of the maxilla. In chapter "Risk Factors" root shape was identified as a risk factor. In three dimensions it is not so clear what an abnormal root shape looks like, and furthermore in most post-treatment images considerably more root damage is visible, especially vertical damage.

Quantification of EARR in 3D brings intriguing possibilities; it is now possible to quantify surface area as well as root volume. These variables may become more important indicators of EARR than the simple point-to-point or point-to-line linear

Fig. 8 CBCT of the maxilla optimized to render the dentition and surrounding bone. Note the wide variation of root shape among the incisors and canines. This makes three-dimensional classification of root shape problematic

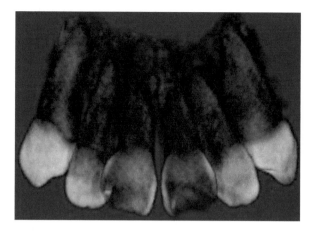

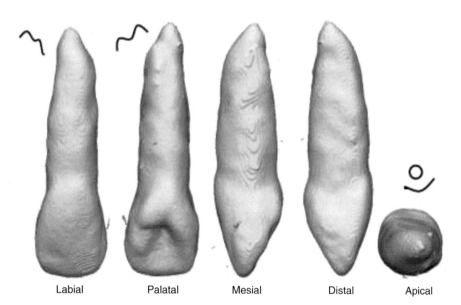

| Labial | Palatal | Mesial | Distal | Apical |

Fig. 9 Segmented maxillary lateral incisor obtained from initial CBCT as part of a study classifying root shape in three dimensions (Clayton 2019). In three dimensions a "step" at the apex was often found which narrowed the root apex. Also note the facial inclination toward the apex—it was also found that the root shape is irregular and asymmetric as it narrows from cervical to apical

measurements used commonly today. Segmentation of the roots is very time consuming and impractical, but improvements in technology will eventually automate the process. Investigating root shape in 3D using segmented teeth is in its infancy but also shows great promise (Ahlbrecht et al. 2017), and see Fig. 9 from Clayton (2019).

4   Measuring Root Displacement

Traditionally root displacement was measured using pre- and post-treatment super-imposed cephalometric films usually employing maxillary superimposition on structures mandated by the American Board of Orthodontics or established methods (Kaley and Phillips 1991; Mirabella and Artun 1995; Linge and Linge 1991; Sameshima and Sinclair 2001). Because the roots of the incisors often obscured one another, assumptions had to be made regarding which root was being measured. Measurement error was therefore high. Apical displacement is one of the main risk factors, but accurate and precise measurement remains elusive, even with high-quality CBCT images. There are three methods of superimposition ((1) point-based, (2) surface-based, (3) voxel-based) all have their advantages and disadvantages, but they share the major limitation of systematic error which is based on both voxel size of the volume, and for the assessment of apical displacement, the resolution of the "fit" of the superimposition which remains too large for the small distances the apex moves (Dang 2017).

5   Summary

Much of the work done in the past using 2D images is being replicated using CBCT images. Visualization of the root is improving rapidly without increasing the patient to higher levels of ionizing radiation (Fig. 10). Smarter algorithms in reconstructing information from DICOM and STL files producing smoother segmentation of specific teeth combined with an accurate surface superimposition algorithm will finally give the clinician and scientist the best data possible. In the meantime, either traditional but digital 2D images are sufficient or 3D renderings equally diagnostic. Clinically, severe EARR is of the most concern, and that can be seen on almost any

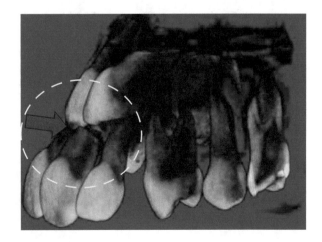

Fig. 10 Pretreatment CBCT of the maxilla clearly shows the extent of root resorption of the maxillary central incisors by the impacted canines. The process of visualization of 3D images is dynamic rather than static as shown by this screen shot; movement of the structures in all three planes of space is easily learned and mastered

image. Figures 11, 12, 13, 14, 15, 16, 17, 18, and 19 summarizes the principles discussed in this chapter.

Case 1

Comparing the panoramic film taken at the same time as the periapical films, all non-digital radiographs. Although the detail is good on the panoramic film, subtle details at the root apices are found on the periapicals of the maxillary lateral incisors showing not only the extent of EARR but the pattern.

The patient was a 39-year-old Hispanic male with chief complaint "I have always wanted to get my smile fixed." He presented with a mild skeletal Class II

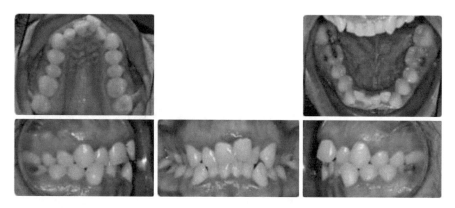

Fig. 11 Initial facial and dental images

Fig. 12 Initial ceph and tracing

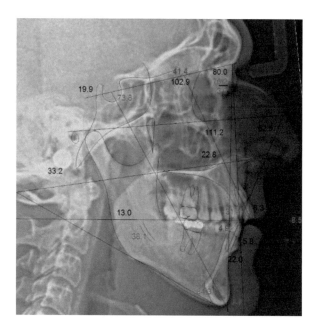

Fig. 13 Initial PAN

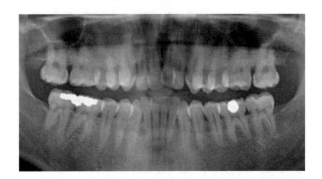

Fig. 14 Initial CBCT

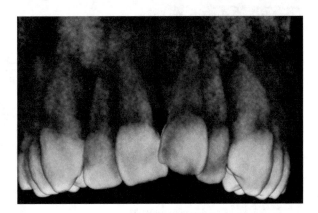

Fig. 15 Progress PAN
after completion of SARPE

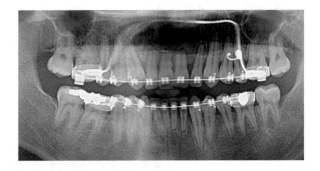

malocclusion characterized by a moderate crowding in both arches and a transverse discrepancy resulting in a posterior bilateral crossbite due to an extremely narrow maxilla (Fig. 11). He had a convex profile, obtuse nasolabial angle, (Fig. 12), but good smile esthetics including incisor show and width. His palatal vault is high, but his uvula and soft palate are normal. Radiographic evaluation was unremarkable with congenitally missing eights by report (Fig. 13). The patient's medical history is non-contributory. He has no current dental problems but has a history of

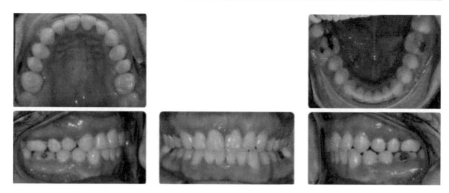

Fig. 16 Final facial and dental images

Fig. 17 Final PAN shows no further EARR except generalized rounding of the apices of all teeth. The combination of EARR and periodontal bone loss will require close monitoring by all dentists taking care of the patient

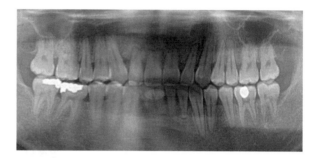

periodontitis treated for many years with conservative scaling and root planning. He appears to have no hard risk factors for EARR.

The treatment plan was to surgically expand the maxilla (SARPE) to create space and correct the transverse problems. In addition to the initial standard orthodontic records, a CBCT was taken (Fig. 14). No periapical x-rays were taken.

Treatment Summary

The progress panoramic radiograph taken after SARPE stabilization (Fig. 15) showed 4–5 mm EARR on the maxillary central incisors and right lateral incisor. Treatment was stopped for 4 months (see chapter "Long-term Prognosis of EARR").

Total treatment time was 38 months. The occlusion is not finished well, and the transverse problem is relapsing (Fig. 16). The maxillary incisor apex was extruded 1.2 mm and displaced palatally 1.0 mm (Fig. 18). Because of the severe EARR visible on the final panoramic image (Fig. 17) and the CBCT (Fig. 19), treatment was terminated. The patient was very happy with the outcome and thoroughly informed about the prognosis of his teeth.

Summary: this case illustrates many of the principles from this chapter and chapter "Risk Factors". Although RME is generally not considered a risk factor, maxillary surgery is. The risk of tooth loss from short roots is discussed in the next chapter.

Fig. 18 Superimposition
of maxilla to show root
apex
displacement—1.2 mm
extrusion and 1.0 mm
palatal movement

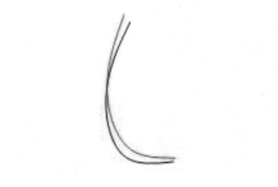

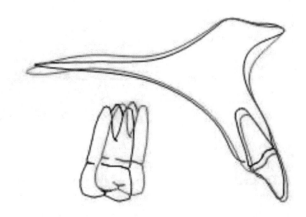

Fig. 19 Final CBCT
clearly shows the extent of
the EARR. This view was
created such that the facial
surfaces of the crowns of
the incisors are exactly
parallel to the page. There
is no distortion in
the image

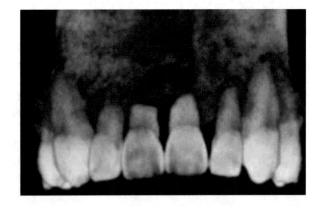

References

Ahlbrecht CA, Ruellas ACO, Paniagua B, Schilling JA, McNamara JA Jr, Cevidanes LHS. Three-dimensional characterization of root morphology for maxillary incisors. PLoS One. 2017;12(6):e0178728.

Christell H, Birch S, Bondemark L, Horner K, Lindh C, SEDENTEXCT Consortium. The impact of cone beam CT on financial costs and orthodontists' treatment decisions in the management of maxillary canines with eruption disturbance. Eur J Orthod. 2018;40(1):65–73.

Clayton C. Classification of 3D maxillary incisor root shape. MS thesis, University of Southern California, Los Angeles, CA; 2019.

Dang N. 3D superimpositions in orthodontics: a review of current techniques and applications. MS thesis, University of Southern California, Los Angeles, CA; 2017.

Hecht R. Root shape frequency and direction of dilaceration: a CBCT study. MS thesis. University of Southern California, Los Angeles; 2013.

Kaley J, Phillips C. Factors related to root resorption in edgewise practice. Angle Orthod. 1991;61:125–32.

Kumar V, Gossett L, Blattner A, Iwasaki LR, Williams K, Nickel JC. Comparison between cone-beam computed tomography and intraoral digital radiography for assessment of tooth root lesions. Am J Orthod Dentofac Orthop. 2011;139(6):e533–41.

Lund H, Gröndahl K, Gröndahl HG. Cone beam computed tomography for assessment of root length and marginal bone level during orthodontic treatment. Angle Orthod. 2010;80(3):466–73.

Mirabella AD, Artun J. Risk factors for apical root resorption of maxillary anterior teeth in adult orthodontic patients. Am J Orthod Dentofac Orthop. 1995;108(1):48–55.

Nakajima A, Sameshima GT, Arai Y, Homme Y, Shimizu N, Dougherty H Sr. Two- and three-dimensional orthodontic imaging using limited cone beam-computed tomography. Angle Orthod. 2005;75(6):895–903.

Peck JL, Sameshima GT, Miller A, Worth P, Hatcher DC. Mesiodistal root angulation using panoramic and cone beam CT. Angle Orthod. 2007;77(2):206–13.

Samandara A, Papageorgiou SN, Ioannidou-Marathiotou I, Kavvadia-Tsatala S, Papadopoulos MA. Evaluation of orthodontically induced external root resorption following orthodontic treatment using cone beam computed tomography (CBCT): a systematic review and meta-analysis. Eur J Orthod. 2019;41(1):67–79.

Sameshima GT, Asgarifar KO. Assessment of root resorption and root shape: periapical vs panoramic films. Angle Orthod. 2001;71(3):185–9.

Sameshima GT, Sinclair PM. Predicting and preventing root resorption: part II. Treatment factors. Am J Orthod Dentofac Orthop. 2001;119(5):511–5.

Sameshima GT, Sinclair PM. Characteristics of patients with severe root resorption. Orthod Craniofac Res. 2004;7(2):108–14.

Walker L, Enciso R, Mah J. Three-dimensional localization of maxillary canines with cone-beam computed tomography. Am J Orthod Dentofac Orthop. 2005;128(4):418–23.

Management

Glenn T. Sameshima

1 Before Treatment Starts

1.1 Thorough History and Good Images

A famous dental malpractice attorney in San Francisco once said "the three R's of malpractice are records, records, records." No truer words were ever spoken. Management of EARR starts with excellent records, such as Standard American Board of Orthodontics records. High-resolution low radiation digital radiographs are preferred—see chapter "Root Resorption". Adults should have a complete periodontal charting.

History: a careful history is essential. This includes dental, medical, and other histories such as did a family relation have any problems with orthodontics. If a patient is at higher risk, specific documentation of this should be included in the informed consent for treatment—see below.

1.2 Informed Consent

The doctrine of informed consent is very important and an essential part of the doctor-patient relationship. It is no different with the risk of EARR. In the United States, the legal/standard of care requires this, and professional associations such as the American Association of Orthodontists and the California Association of Orthodontists provide this for their members—see Fig. 1. Additionally, management of EARR should include an informed patient regarding the risks and the possibility that treatment goals cannot be met and that there will be a need and cost of more frequent periapical or panoramic radiographs. For patients who have higher

G. T. Sameshima (✉)
Advanced Orthodontics, Herman Ostrow School of Dentistry of the University of Southern California, Los Angeles, CA, USA
e-mail: sameshim@usc.edu

© Springer Nature Switzerland AG 2021
G. T. Sameshima (ed.), *Clinical Management of Orthodontic Root Resorption*,
https://doi.org/10.1007/978-3-030-58706-2_7

problem, the
ient cooperation.
/ close to the
ment may be
pated growth
the dentofacial
ental problems
ot adequate.
eatment plan
nt time is extend-
ditional fees may

can expect an
nfort due to
ances. Non-
used during

oes not guaran-
est of vour life

without of thouontic treatment, but the risk is greater
to an individual wearing braces or other appliances.
These problems may be aggravated if the patient
has not had the benefit of fluoridated water or its
substitute, or if the patient consumes sweetened
beverages or foods.

Root Resorption
The roots of some patients' teeth become shorter
(resorption) during orthodontic treatment. It is not
known exactly what causes root resorption, nor is it
possible to predict which patients will experience it.
However, many patients have retained teeth through-
out life with severely shortened roots. If resorption
is detected during orthodontic treatment, your
orthodontist may recommend a pause in treatment
or the removal of the appliances prior to the completion of orthodontic treatment.

Nerve Damage
A tooth that has been traumatized by an accident or
deep decay may have experienced damage to the
nerve of the tooth. Orthodontic tooth movement may,

mandibular join
ear problems. I
the jaw joints, i
head or face), ɛ
joint problems,
poorly balancec
Jaw joint proble
dontic treatmer
pain, jaw poppi
should be prom
Treatment by o
may be necess

Impacted, ɪ Unerupted
Teeth may beco
or gums), ankyl
to erupt. Oftent
apparent reasoɪ
Treatment of th
ular circumstan
involved tooth, ɛ
exposure, surgiɪ

Fig. 1 Root resorption paragraph from sample informed consent document

risk, it is recommended that a more specific documented conversation be noted in
the chart and acknowledged by the patient.

1.3   Staff and Referring Doctors

Office staff, both front and back must be aware of all risks of dental treatment.
This is akin to education about why good oral hygiene is so important. Patients
often ask staff questions they feel reluctant to ask the doctor. Staff must be able to
answer questions about EARR truthfully and accurately. Many dentists do not know
much about orthodontic root resorption and do not understand that long-term risk
of tooth loss is not high even for a tooth that is severely resorbed (see next chapter).
Misunderstandings about the cause of EARR can lead to unnecessary expenditure
of time and resources for the dentist and the patient.

2   During Active Treatment

2.1   Before Finishing Stages

For patients not at higher risk: it is good practice to document with progress
records minimally a PAN and a thorough check up with the general dentist. When

does EARR start? Artun has shown that if EARR is found in the first 6–12 months of treatment, then the affected teeth are at risk for further EARR (Artun et al. 2005). This supports the rationale for progress radiographs.

What Do I Do if I See EARR at Progress?

If progress films show active EARR of greater than 2 mm, then the orthodontist must decide whether or not to continue moving the affected teeth. IF EARR equals 3 mm or more (less if the root is short to begin with), then treatment must be halted for 4 months. Four months is the length of the *human bone remodeling cycle*; for approximately 1 month, osteoclast activity is gradually replaced by a 3-month period of repair. The surface remodels and so does the root apex; however, there is no deposition or replacement of the lost cementum at the apex. During this quiescent period, the root surface and apex, as well as the lamina dura and periodontal ligament, return to the biologic and physiologic state of equilibrium they were in before orthodontic tooth movement was started. It has been shown that resuming treatment is without increased risk. The clinician must explain the delay to the patient and obtain their consent (and document it). Patients are usually understanding about the delay if the dentist is forthright and sympathetic.

The case shown in Figs. 2, 3, 4, 5, 6, and 7 illustrates management of EARR mid-treatment. The patient presented with a Class I malocclusion characterized by crowding, convex profile, and proclined incisors with poor facial esthetics (Figs. 2, 3, and 4). The treatment plan was ideal incisor goals consistent with good facial esthetics by extracting four bicuspids. Appliance was a 0.022 SWA. Treatment was prolonged due to missed appointments and broken appliances. Progress records were taken at 3 years (Fig. 5), and severe and moderate EARR was detected on many teeth, notably the maxillary central incisors. The decision was made to halt treatment for 4 months. Minimal detailing followed, and the case was debanded 6 months after the quiescent stage was finished (Fig. 6). The final PAN shows no further EARR (Fig. 7).

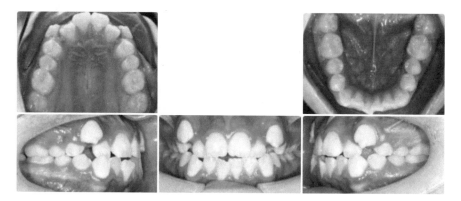

Fig. 2 Initial intraoral images

Fig. 3 Initial
cephalometric tracing

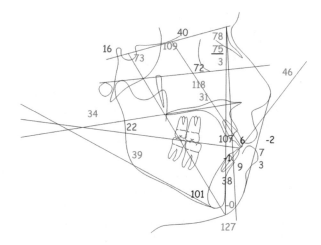

Fig. 4 Initial PAN

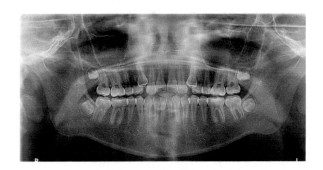

Fig. 5 Progress PAN

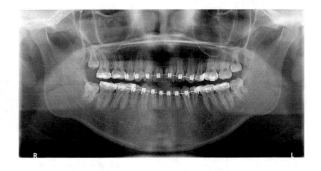

Fig. 6 Final PAN

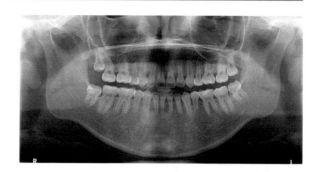

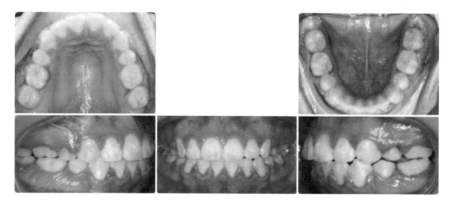

Fig. 7 Final intraoral images

2.2   During Finishing Stages

This decision is similar to EARR before finishing as in the previous paragraph. This decision will be based upon how close to finishing the case is and how much apical displacement is necessary to achieve the desired outcome. Usually if the amount of tooth movement is minimal and the case is close to finishing, then the clinician can proceed but must not prolong treatment unduly and may have to accept compromises in detailing the case. However, if greater movements are required such as torque or space closure, then the recommended strategy is to halt treatment for a minimum of 4 months as described in Sect. 2.1.

If the amount of EARR is 4 mm or more, the patient has been in treatment for a long time, and the apex has already been moved a significant distance (1 mm or more), then the orthodontist has a critical decision—halt treatment and remove the appliances or carefully finish if major problems still remain such as space or poor esthetic positioning of the anterior maxillary incisors). Even if a case is close to finishing, a treatment halt of 4 months can still be done if both dentist and patient agree that the outcomes will be worth it.

In any situation where EARR is found, it cannot be emphasized enough that everyone involved with the patient's care be thoroughly informed.

3   Post-treatment

What do I do if I see EARR at the end of treatment? Post-treatment radiographs should be taken to assess root resorption; obviously if progress radiographs showed EARR, then further progress radiographs would be beneficial. Regardless of the amount of EARR, the orthodontist must inform the patient and the patient's general dentist immediately. Fortunately, EARR ceases when active forces are halted. This physiological process takes approximately 4 weeks. There is no evidence that EARR continues with passive retention, either fixed or removable. The use of spring aligners is probably without harm, but tooth positioners may not. In retention and beyond, there may be radiographic evidence of a rounding of the root apex.

4   Summary

Table 1 summarizes the clinical management of pretreatment and in-progress EARR. Table 2 summarizes the clinical management of post-treatment EARR. In both circumstances, the most important point to remember is educating the patient and any health professionals participating in the patient's care.

Clinical Case 1
Long treatment time—treatment terminated. The records are displayed in Figs. 2, 3, 4, 5, 6, and 7.

The patient is a 14-year-old Hispanic female (Fig. 2). She presented with a Class I malocclusion with severe (12 mm in the maxillary arch with labially blocked

Table 1 Clinical management: pretreatment and progress

1. Good pretreatment images
2. If risk factors present document special entry in informed consent
3. If short roots are present at the beginning of treatment
4. Delay appliances on the affected tooth as long as possible
5. Avoid torque and apical displacement
6. Take more frequent periapicals
7. If risk factors present take periapicals at 6–12 months or when apical displacement has started
8. During treatment:
    (a) If EARR greater than 2 mm stop for 4 months
    (b) If EARR greater than 4 mm or more than one-third of the root stop active tooth movement, consider terminating treatment
9. If severe EARR occurs on more than two adjacent teeth must consider termination of treatment
10. Patient and referring dentist must be kept informed at all-time points

Table 2 Clinical management: post-treatment

1. Good post-treatment images
2. Inform the patient and document
3. Inform the patient's general dentist and other dentists involved with the patient's care (e.g., periodontist)
4. EARR stops when appliances are removed
5. No EARR with retainers of any kind or spring aligners
6. No increased risk for devitalized pulp
7. Root apices will round off over time
8. Splinting usually unnecessary but if more than two teeth affected 4–6 months
9. No increased risk for tooth loss with good oral hygiene
10. If trauma to the teeth – tooth with a short risk possibly have a higher risk for avulsion but not fracture

out canines) crowding, convex profile with lip strain, decalcified teeth, poor oral hygiene, a low frenum, and zero overjet and overbite with the mandibular central incisors and canines in anterior crossbite. Her chief complaint was "crooked, ugly teeth." Cephalometrically she is a Class I skeletal malocclusion, high mandibular plane angle, with protrusive incisors by all analyses with the lower incisor markedly proclined (Fig. 3). There is no history of trauma, airway problems, allergies, or other relevant medical conditions; she is not growing taller and is not taking any medications.

The initial PAN (Fig. 4) reveals developing third molars in all quadrants, long roots in general with occasional mild dilacerations. The root apices are unfortunately indistinct, but length and shape are acceptable.

The proposed treatment was maximum anchorage and extraction of four first premolars. Anchorage included a high-pull headgear and trans palatal bar. The appliance was a 022 straight wire (self-ligation) with a wire sequence of nickel titanium round and rectangular, TMA rectangular, and stainless steel finishing. The patient wore Class II and up and down finishing elastics. Oral hygiene during treatment was problematic, and the patient missed numerous appointments.

The total treatment time was 5 years well beyond the mean for this type of case due to failed appointments and broken appliances. Treatment was halted for hygiene twice but continued. Vertical control of the anterior segment was difficult. No progress radiographs were taken until 4 years into treatment when the canines were finally brought into the arch. Steel wires had been in place for 6 months for torque when the 3-year progress PAN shown in Fig. 5 was finally taken.

The case was discussed with the parents, and a mutual decision was made to end treatment. The final PAN (Fig. 6) taken 1 month after debanding shows generalized EARR with severe EARR occurring for the maxillary central incisors. Each central incisor lost 5 mm resulting in a crown root ratio of less than 50 percent. All 4 s premolars had 4 mm of EARR. The initial PAN did not show any evidence, but the pattern of EARR is highly suggestive of SRA. The patient, parents, and general dentist were all informed of the EARR, its prognosis, and etiology. Final photos are shown in Figure 7.

Four important points from this case:

1. Take progress radiographs!
2. Monitor treatment time.
3. Do not be afraid to STOP treatment.
4. Use caution with up and down anterior elastics—although never proven experimentally, clinicians have long suspected and found that "jiggling" the anterior teeth with vertical elastics worn for a long time with sporadic cooperation can lead to severe EARR. The pattern in this case is not completely consistent with that theory as the lateral incisors were not affected as much. Cephalometric superimposition (not shown) is not useful here either as it showed that the maxillary incisor apex extruded 1 mm and did not move horizontally.

Clinical Case 2
When does EARR stop? (Figs. 8, 9, 10, and 11)

This patient is a 12-year-old Asian female with a chief complaint of "crooked teeth." Her health history and dental history are negative for EARR risk factors, and she does not have any history of deleterious oral habits or trauma to the face or teeth. She has normal height and weight for her age and is still growing.

Clinically she has dentoalveolar protrusion with lip strain and mild crowding and rotated anterior teeth. Overjet and overbite are normal. Facial esthetics—midlines, smile arc, etc.—are acceptable.

Cephalometrically she presented with a skeletal Class II Division I malocclusion—ANB = 6 with mandibular retrusion (SNB = 75). Incisors are protrusive (Steiner 7 mm at 30° and 10 mm at 37°).

- Interincisal = 106
- IMPA = 102
- Mx 1 to SN = 111
- Thin biotype

Dilacerated, irregular root shape and mesiodens near the apex of #9

Fig. 8 Initial PAN for Clinical Case 2

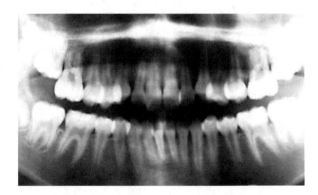

Fig. 9 Initial periapicals

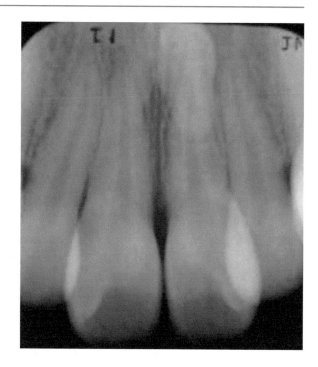

Fig. 10 Final periapicals

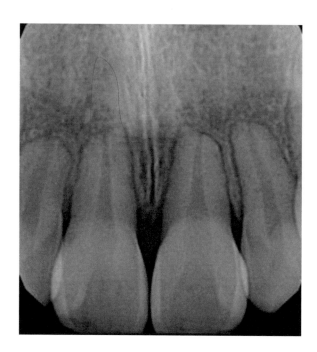

Fig. 11 Six months post
appliance removal. No
further EARR is noted

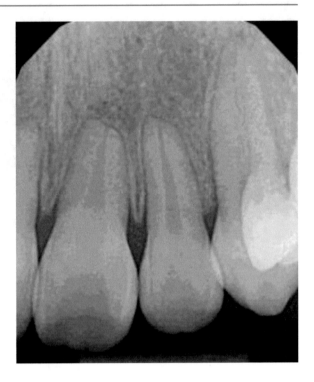

Outcome: after 6 months in retention, the general dentist took new periapicals. It is clear that the EARR has stopped completely with no further root shortening. Periodontal examination found no mobility. Retention with Hawleys was continued full time.

5   Retreatment

Occasionally patients decide not to wear their retainers as instructed, and teeth relapse. These patients may have experienced EARR during their treatment, and now they present with short roots. This situation is no different from the patient who never had orthodontics treatment who also has short roots. See previous sections and chapter "Risk Factors". If all four maxillary incisors have lost more than half the root length (by report, by available pre- and post-treatment periapicals (best), or estimation), then the following is a good way to proceed:

1. Make sure the patient finished orthodontic treatment 12 months ago.
2. Make sure the patient understands that the short roots could get even shorter, but studies show root shortening does not necessarily mean you will lose the teeth.
3. Get #2 in writing or record it.

4. Don't use any rectangular wire and get the brackets on perfect the first time (avoid tweaking).
5. Get in and out ASAP.
6. Bond 3-3 Zachrisson style when done (unless you are pretty sure the teeth won't move, then use a Hawley or Essix).
7. Make sure the patient's restorative dentist knows.

Treatment Options

Glenn T. Sameshima

The key to understanding treatment options lies in understanding risk factors, educating the patient and dentist, and determining the best plan for the patient. This may involve compromises or alternative plans. Justus (2015) stated that there were five ways to prevent or circumvent EARR:

1. Growth modification to correct severe skeletal Class II malocclusions
2. Early interception of maxillary canines that have mesial eruption paths
3. Serial extraction to modify eruption paths (guidance of eruption)
4. Correction of anterior open bite with a palatal tongue spur appliance
5. Orthognathic surgery to avoid moving teeth large distances and against cortical plates

Growth modification would prevent the need to extract teeth and/or displace the maxillary incisor roots palatally and distally. The second two strategies would decrease the chances of an erupting maxillary canine damaging the root of the lateral incisor. Correction of anterior open bite if caused by tongue posture is certainly a practical treatment regardless, but if the open bite is skeletal, then intrusion of the posterior segments using skeletal anchorage is a superior approach. And correcting skeletal problems with orthognathic surgery instead of "camouflage" is also excellent advice especially if the patient has EARR risk factors. However, the caveat in Chapter 5 regarding surgery of the maxilla must also be understood.

We propose the following as general rules of engagement when confronted with patients with risk factors. Most clinicians are most concerned about maxillary incisors with short roots before treatment even starts.

G. T. Sameshima (✉)
Advanced Orthodontics, Herman Ostrow School of Dentistry of the University of Southern California, Los Angeles, CA, USA
e-mail: sameshim@usc.edu

© Springer Nature Switzerland AG 2021
G. T. Sameshima (ed.), *Clinical Management of Orthodontic Root Resorption*,
https://doi.org/10.1007/978-3-030-58706-2_8

1. No treatment
2. No appliances on at-risk teeth
3. Avoid root movement
4. Short treatment time
5. Limited objectives
6. Extractions and Implants

1   No Treatment

Sometimes the best treatment is no treatment or no orthodontics. Veneers or other restorative solutions may be preferred. Extraction of short-rooted teeth in itself is not a justification for implants; however, in certain situations it may be the best course.

2   No Appliances on At-Risk Teeth

Do not band or bond any brackets or attachments on teeth at high risk, if possible for the treatment entirety, if not then for as long as necessary for alignment and space closure. Brackets must be placed precisely, so no tweaking with wire bends or repositioning becomes necessary.

3   Avoid Root Movement

The orthodontist must limit apical displacement including torque and bodily movement. Rotation and tipping on a limited basis with no round tripping is acceptable. Patient must be forewarned for the need of more frequent radiographs.

4   Short Treatment Time

Treatment time must not exceed the normal treatment duration for the type of case. Treatment goals may have to be compromised. Patients' cooperation in not missing appointments or breaking appliances is important. Oral hygiene must be monitored and appropriate steps taken.

5   Limited Objectives

Treatment goals must be changed or adjusted as described by Justus above. Limited goals must be considered to minimize exaggerated tooth movement of at-risk teeth. If comprehensive full treatment is done, the patient must acknowledge the risks—see Chap. 7 management.

6 Extractions and Implants

Extraction cases generally take longer, but with proper mechanics and minimizing movement of at-risk teeth, extractions for moderate to severe crowding can be managed. Judicious IPR should be considered. Not achieving ideal or desired outcomes even such as correcting overjet and overbite completely must be an acceptable compromise, and the patient must be so informed. An interesting solution was presented by Carlier et al. (2019) in which "surgery first" of the lower jaw (and en bloc osteotomies) were performed on a 14-year-old patient who had idiopathic root resorption.

7 Endodontic Therapy and EARR

Clinical experience and the orthodontic (and endodontic) literature tend to support the finding that endodontically treated teeth do not get EARR. Bender et al. reported this in 1997 with a case series review (43 patients). In their comprehensive study of over 1000 patients, Sameshima and Sinclair (2001) found no EARR in teeth that had had a root canal. Spurrier et al. 1990 and Mirabella and Artun 1995 reported similar findings. A systematic review (Walker 2010) was inconclusive due to a lack of randomized clinical trials. Resorption of the root apex was found in endodontically treated maxillary incisors after orthodontic tooth movement in a split mouth study, but there was no significant difference (Llamas-Carreras et al. 2012). Kolcuoğlu and Oz (2020) found significantly less EARR in a split mouth design; a previous split mouth study (Lee and Lee 2016) also found less to no EARR in the root filled teeth compared to the contralateral vital controls.

8 Early Treatment

Two-phase treatment. The proportion of incisors with moderate to severe EARR was slightly greater in the single phase treatment group than a cohort of two-phase patients Brin et al. (2003). The risk of developing EARR 41% lower in two-phase orthodontic treatment was reported recently (Fernandes et al. 2019). Not factored in was maturity of the apex and distance teeth were moved. Teeth with immature apices do not normally resorb (Mavragani et al. 2002)—see the Chapter 3 "Etiology" in this book for the possible mechanism. One unpublished thesis (Do 2002) found that a small proportion of roots may not achieve their full length if moved orthodontically, but generally an immature apex seems to have a protective effect. Peg and small laterals do not have a higher risk (Kook et al. 2003).

Preventing root resorption caused by erupting canines or other impacted teeth. It is well documented that maxillary lateral incisors are often damaged by erupting canines, ectopic, or normal. EARR is indirectly affected if other factors induce EARR during orthodontic tooth movement. Details are provided in Chapter 10; however, the clinician can take some steps to avoid root damage if they suspect a canine is erupting too close to the lateral root or is on an eruption pathway that will bring it too close (Schroder et al. 2018; Grybienė et al. 2019). (1) Take a good limited CBCT. Bjerklin in 2006 in a study of 113 retained maxillary canines in children showed that the addition of a CT scan to traditional initial orthodontic records changed the treatment plan in 44% of the cases mostly because the 3D image showed more damage on some teeth and less damage on other teeth! (2) Extract primary maxillary canines early. (3) Expand the arch with RME in addition to extracting primary canines if there is insufficient arch length.

Let us examine a case that illustrates several points brought up in this chapter and previous ones (Figs. 1, 2, 3, and 4):

The patient is a 13-year-old boy who has a chief complaint of a "fang tooth." He and his family are anxious to start treatment. No one in their family has ever had orthodontic treatment of any type. He has no history of trauma, oral habits, or significant dental or medical problems, although he has had minimal exposure to both. He has a convex profile, and his teeth are protrusive with lip strain. Cephalometrically he has mild bimaxillary protrusion with a skeletal Class I jaw relationship. His dental midlines are on, and both arches are crowded. The maxillary right lateral incisor

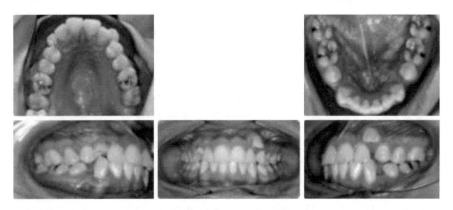

Fig. 1 Initial records—intraoral

Fig. 2 Initial PAN

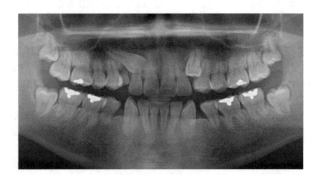

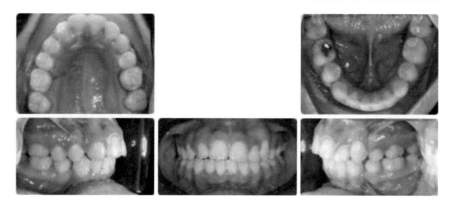

Fig. 3 Final intraoral images

Fig. 4 Final PAN

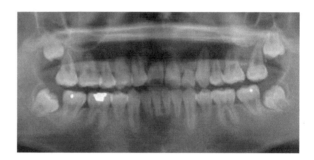

appears to be missing, and the left maxillary canine is completely blocked out. He is also missing two mandibular bicuspids. His right first molar through to the right canine is in crossbite with the mandibular teeth (Fig. 1). The ABO Discrepancy Index is greater than 20. He has multiple teeth with short roots, most notably the maxillary central incisors and all four second bicuspids. The maxillary left lateral incisor has a damaged root from the erupting canine (Fig. 2).

Precautions?
(a) Avoid long treatment time.
(b) Do not displace the apices of the incisors and second bicuspids very far—avoid heavy torque.

Treatment Options?
(a) No orthodontics—extract the maxillary left canine and send him on his way!
(b) Orthodontics—extract the maxillary lateral incisor and one lower incisor.
(c) Orthodontics—extract three bicuspids for crowding and profile
(d) Orthodontics—canines to Class I (extract four bicuspids), create ideal space for the maxillary incisors with plans to extract the three teeth and replace them with four implants for his 21st birthday.

After much head-scratching, the orthodontist decided to extract three bicuspids and do a canine substitution for the missing maxillary right lateral incisor. The patient's parents were informed of the possibility that his teeth could get shorter in order to obtain the desired results. Fixed appliances were placed from the beginning on all teeth. Rectangular 16×22 wires were the largest stiffest wires used in treatment. Progress PANs were taken twice. At 18 months the PAN showed EARR. Treatment was stopped and appliances removed (Fig. 3 (intraoral images) and 4 (PAN)).

References

Bender IB, Byers MR, Mori K. Periapical replacement resorption of permanent, vital, endodontically treated incisors after orthodontic movement: report of two cases. J Endod. 1997;23(12):768–73.

Bjerklin K, Ericson S. How a computerized tomography examination changed the treatment plans of 80 children with retained and ectopically positioned maxillary canines. Angle Orthod. 2006;76(1):43–51.

Brin I, Tulloch JF, Koroluk L, Phillips C. External apical root resorption in Class II malocclusion: a retrospective review of 1- versus 2-phase treatment. Am J Orthod Dentofac Orthop. 2003;124(2):151–6.

Carlier A, Van de Casteele E, Van Erum R, Nadjmi N. Orthodontic -surgical management in a Class II case with idiopathic root resorption. J Stomatol Oral Maxillofac Surg. 2019;120(3):263–6.

Do PT. The effect of orthodontic tooth movement on premolar root development. MS thesis. University of Southern California, Los Angeles; 2002.

Fernandes LQP, Figueiredo NC, Montalvany Antonucci CC, Lages EMB, Andrade I Jr, Capelli Junior J. Predisposing factors for external apical root resorption associated with orthodontic treatment. Korean J Orthod. 2019;49(5):310–8.

Grybienė V, Juozėnaitė D, Kubiliūtė K. Diagnostic methods and treatment strategies of impacted maxillary canines: a literature review. Stomatologija. 2019;21(1):3–12.

Justus R. Prevention of orthodontic root resorption. In: Iatrogenic effects of orthodontic treatment: decision-making in prevention, diagnosis, and treatment; 2015.

Kolcuoğlu K, Oz AZ. Comparison of orthodontic root resorption of root-filled and vital teeth using micro-computed tomography. Angle Orthod. 2020;90(1):56–62.

Kook YA, Park S, Sameshima GT. Peg-shaped and small lateral incisors not at higher risk for root resorption. Am J Orthod Dentofac Orthop. 2003;123(3):253–8.

Lee YJ, Lee TY. External root resorption during orthodontic treatment in root-filled teeth and contralateral teeth with vital pulp: a clinical study of contributing factors. Am J Orthod Dentofac Orthop. 2016;149(1):84–91.

Llamas-Carreras JM, Amarilla A, Espinar-Escalona E, Castellanos-Cosano L, Martín-González J, Sánchez-Domínguez B, López-Frías FJ. External apical root resorption in maxillary root-filled incisors after orthodontic treatment: a split-mouth design study. Med Oral Patol Oral Cir Bucal. 2012;17(3):e523–7.

Mavragani M, Boe OE, Wisth PJ, Selvig KA. Changes in root length during orthodontic treatment: advantages for immature teeth. Eur J Orthod. 2002;24:91–7.

Mirabella AD, Artun J. Risk factors for apical root resorption of maxillary anterior teeth in adult orthodontic patients. Am J Orthod Dentofac Orthop. 1995;108(1):48–55.

Sameshima GT, Sinclair PM. Predicting and preventing root resorption: Part II. Treatment factors. Am J Orthod Dentofac Orthop. 2001;119(5):511–5.

Schroder AGD, Guariza-Filho O, de Araujo CM, Ruellas AC, Tanaka OM, Porporatti AL. To what extent are impacted canines associated with root resorption of the adjacent tooth?: A systematic review with meta-analysis. J Am Dent Assoc. 2018;149(9):765–77.

Spurrier SW, Hall SH, Joondeph DR, Shapiro PA, Riedel RA. A comparison of apical root resorption during orthodontic treatment in endodontically treated and vital teeth. Am J Orthod Dentofac Orthop. 1990;97(2):130–4.

Walker, S. Root resorption during orthodontic treatment. Evid Based Dent. 2010;11:88.

Long-term Prognosis of EARR

Glenn T. Sameshima

1 Introduction

Perhaps the most important chapter in this book for the clinician! Orthodontists in particular find the occurrence of significant root-shortening disquieting. See previous chapter. Is a tooth with a short root at higher risk of being lost simply by virtue of a short root? Does crown-root ratio make any difference? Does the age of a patient have anything to do with prognosis? Function or parafunction? Health of the patient? What if more than one tooth is affected? The good news is that the answer is that NO, the tooth is NOT at increased risk to be lost!

2 Basis for Favorable Long-term Prognosis

As any reasonably trained dentist should realize, the overriding factor in determining the long-term longevity of any tooth is the health of the periodontium. Periodontists have always regarded orthodontists with puzzlement with the latter's worry that the teeth with short roots will be lost sooner than they should be. Biologically and physiologically, a tooth with a healthy periodontium should outlast the body it is attached to regardless of root length! In fact, as humans age there is a gradual increase in the thickness of cementum surrounding the root apex (not to be confused with the occurrence of a cementoma, a pathological condition). Hypercementosis is an aberrant form of this deposition of cementum in the aging human. This fact is well-documented, and anthropologists and scientists from other disciplines actually use this information to estimate the age of a person by counting the number of cementum "rings" from a root, analogous to estimating the age of trees based on counting the rings in the tree trunk (Gupta et al. 2014). Root surface

G. T. Sameshima (✉)
Advanced Orthodontics, Herman Ostrow School of Dentistry of the University of Southern California, Los Angeles, CA, USA
e-mail: sameshim@usc.edu

© Springer Nature Switzerland AG 2021
G. T. Sameshima (ed.), *Clinical Management of Orthodontic Root Resorption*,
https://doi.org/10.1007/978-3-030-58706-2_9

area for the apical third of a tooth contributes very little to the periodontal support of the tooth due to the three dimensional geometry of the root (Consolaro 2019).

3   Long-term Prognosis: Literature

The real question here is what is the prognosis of any tooth that has a short root? Secondarily, does EARR from orthodontic tooth movement have a different prognosis from teeth that are congenitally short? The answer to the second question is no, there is no difference in fate between a tooth with a short root from orthodontics and a tooth that has a naturally short root. The following paragraphs answer the first question.

What is the evidence? If we look at clinical experience, the majority of orthodontists and dentists will probably admit that they never saw a tooth lost just because it had a short root, trauma and periodontal disease notwithstanding. Falahat et al. (2008) looked at 32 resorbed incisors (from erupting canines) several years later. They found that 13 of the teeth had undergone repair naturally, 12 were unchanged, and in 7 teeth further resorption had taken place. None of the teeth were in danger of being lost. Becker and Chaushu (2005) found that maxillary lateral incisors with severe root resorption (not apical) caused by erupting canines could be moved orthodontically. In that study, teeth that had EARR such that a 20% increase in crown root ratio occurred were still stable long term.

Generally, there seems to be no real relationship between teeth with EARR and their loss long term, according to case reports and long-term cohort studies. Remington et al. (1989) recalled 100 patients who had EARR from orthodontic treatment 14 years later and found that no teeth had been compromised. Savage and Kokich Sr. (2002) presented three cases that were recalled many years after treatment that had had severe EARR of the maxillary incisors. They found no further problems but emphasized the need for an interdisciplinary approach to maintain the teeth long term. Another study (Jönsson et al. 2007) recalled patients who had significant EARR 25 years later. They found significantly more tooth mobility if the tooth length was less than 9 mm, but no greater risk. Marques et al. (2011) reported a case in which there was severe EARR of all four maxillary incisors from orthodontic treatment; the case was stable 25 years later with no further EARR or other problems. In chapter 10 "Resorption of Impacted Teeth" the fate of maxillary lateral incisors with damaged roots from canine eruption is discussed, but briefly, such teeth can still safely be moved orthodontically and are stable long term (Bjerklin and Guitirokh 2011). However, a long-term, prospective study following patients with EARR has not been accomplished yet; this would be illuminating indeed.

Teeth with short roots, regardless of the reason (congenital or EARR), do not have greater morbidity and unless there are active, untreated periodontal problems will not fall out one day. The success of dental implants may influence a minority of restorative dentists to wrongly replace a healthy tooth with a short root with extraction and an implant. Once 6 months have passed in retention, teeth stabilize, including those with short roots, as long as they are not in hyperfunction. However, compared to a tooth with a long root, obviously a tooth with a short root has a greater chance of being avulsed if impacted directly by a traumatic event like a fist or steering wheel. It has been suggested that persons with short-rooted maxillary incisors have been even more cognizant by wearing mouth guards in athletics, but there are no RCTs that have tested this measure.

Three clinical cases illustrate these principles: Figs. 1, 2, 3, 4, 5, 6, 7, 8, 9, 10, 11, 12, 13, and 14. Figure 15 follows up the case from Chapter 5 "Risk Factors"—4 years after debanding.

Fig. 1 Case 1: Initial PAN

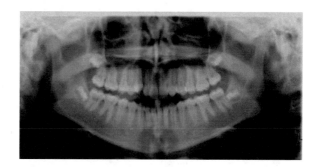

Fig. 2 Case 1: Final PAN—generalized moderate to severe EARR. The patient and general dentist were immediately informed and the etiology and prognosis discussed and documented. At the 6-month retainer check, there was NO tooth mobility

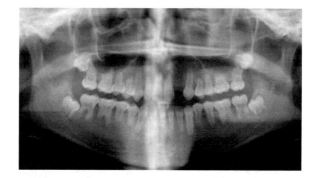

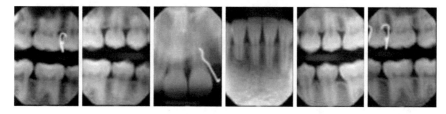

Fig. 3 Case 1: Four years after appliance removal. There is no further EARR, and teeth and orthodontic result is very stable. Patient is still wearing her "flipper"

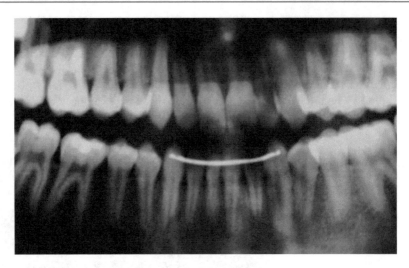

Fig. 4 Case 2: Post-treatment PAN day of appliance removal

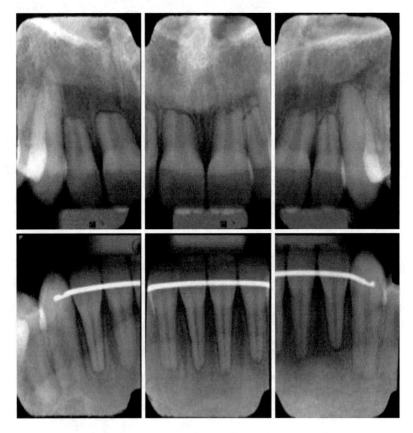

Fig. 5 Case 2: Periapical radiographs taken 7 years after appliance removal

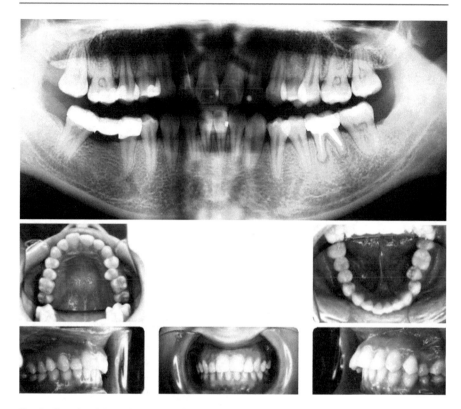

Fig. 6 Case 3: Initial radiographs and extraoral images

Fig. 7 Case 3: Progress 1 Right = one year. Progress 2 Left = one month prior to debonding

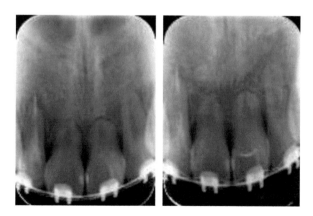

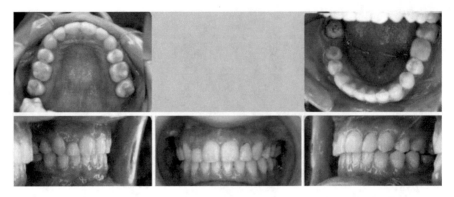

Fig. 8 Case 3: Final intraoral images

Fig. 9 Case 3: Six months post-treatment

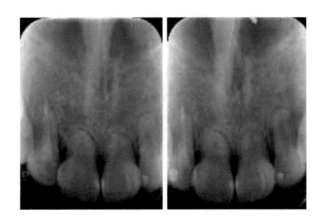

Fig. 10 Case 3: Two years post-treatment

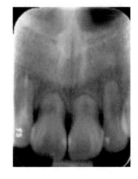

Clinical Case 1

Figures 1, 2, 3. The patient was in fine health with no predisposing factors. She was 15.3 years old at the start of treatment. The chief complaint was "underbite." She presented with a skeletal Class I malocclusion and anterior crossbite. The maxillary left lateral incisor is congenitally missing. The midlines were off. The

Fig. 11 Case 3: Three years post -treatment

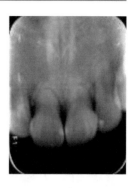

Fig. 12 Case 3: Four
years post-treatment

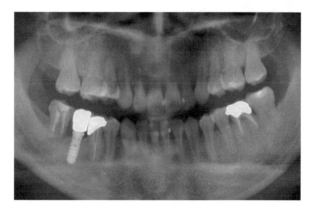

treatment plan was to create implant space for the missing tooth and flare the maxillary incisors to correct the anterior crossbite. The patient completed non-extraction orthodontic therapy with 0.022 SWA for 28 months. Cooperation with Class III and midline elastics was good.

Clinical Case 2
Patient had 30 months of orthodontic treatment with fixed appliances. All four maxillary incisors had severe EARR (Fig. 4). The PAN and periapical radiographs in Figure 5 were taken 7 years after treatment. Patient reports no symptoms. Teeth are not mobile. There is no further EARR.

Clinical Case 3
Initial records (Figure 6). 24-year-old Asian female. Chief complaint "I have an overbite and my top front teeth stick out." No history of previous orthodontic treatment. Excess overjet and deep bite. Lip strain. Skeletal dental Class II Division 1.

Case 3 Summary
First of all, note the difference in root length seen in the periapicals vs the PAN in the initial stage of treatment. Because the maxillary incisors were so flared, they appear longer as treatment progresses; this is due to increasing lingual tip. At the end of

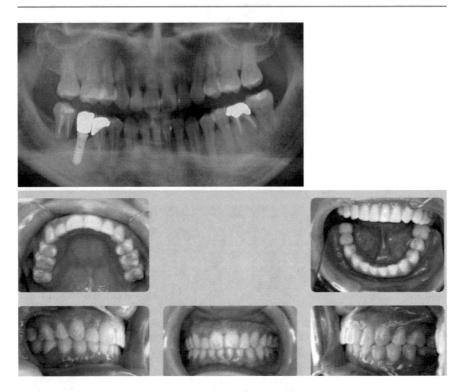

Fig. 13 Case 3: Six years post-treatment. Final intraoral images

Fig. 14 Case 3: Eight years post-treatment

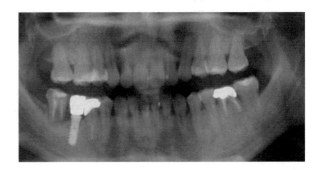

treatment, EARR was approximately 3 mm for both maxillary incisors. There was no further EARR at all-time points post-retention (Figures 8–13). Teeth were stable with no mobility. Eight-year recall (Figure 14) when patient brought her first child in, she was still very pleased with the outcome! She had been counseled about the outcome and shown the pre- and post-treatment radiographs and subsequent follow-up. She saw her general dentist annually, and he duly checked the periodontal condition. The patient said the general dentist was surprised at how stable the teeth were.

Fig. 15 Case 3: Four-year follow-up PAN of patient case in Chapter 5 "Risk Factors" (Clinical Case 8). The adult patient had significant EARR due to extended treatment time and an impacted tooth. There is no further EARR

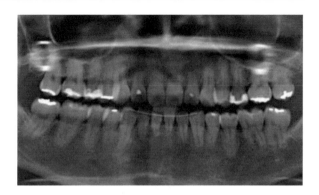

Clinical Case 4

The next case was contributed by Dr. Ernest Jou of Taipei, Taiwan.

This case was presented in chapter 5 "Risk Factors" as an example of EARR due to extended treatment time. There was generalized EARR (rounding of the root apices) and significant EARR in the maxillary incisors. The PAN (Figure 15) taken four years later shows no further EARR, and there were no patient symptoms, and no tooth mobility. The general dentist is aware of the EARR and has reinforced the importance of good oral hygiene for a healthy periodontium. The patient is fully informed and understands that the long-term risk of tooth loss is minimal.

References

Becker A, Chaushu S. Long-term follow-up of severely resorbed maxillary incisors after resolution of an etiologically associated impacted canine. Am J Orthod Dentofac Orthop. 2005;127(6):650–4.

Bjerklin K, Guitirokh CH. Maxillary incisor root resorption induced by ectopic canines. Angle Orthod. 2011;81(5):800–6.

Consolaro A. Extreme root resorption in orthodontic practice: teeth do not have to be replaced with implants. Dental Press J Orthod. 2019;24(5):20–8.

Falahat B, Ericson S, Mak D'Amico R, Bjerklin K. Incisor root resorption due to ectopic maxillary canines: a long-term radiographic follow-up. Angle Orthod. 2008;78(5):778–85.

Gupta P, Kaur H, Shankari GSM, Jawanda MK, Sahi N. Human age estimation from tooth cementum and dentin. J Clin Diagn Res. 2014;8(4):ZC07–10.

Jönsson A, Malmgren O, Levander E. Long-term follow-up of tooth mobility in maxillary incisors with orthodontically induced apical root resorption. Eur J Orthod. 2007;29(5):482–7.

Marques LS, Chaves KC, Rey AC, Pereira LJ, Ruellas AC. Severe root resorption and orthodontic treatment: clinical implications after 25 years of follow-up. Am J Orthod Dentofac Orthop. 2011;139(4 Suppl):S166–9.

Remington DN, Joondeph DR, Artun J, Riedel RA, Chapko MK. Long-term evaluation of root resorption occurring during orthodontic treatment. Am J Orthod Dentofac Orthop. 1989;96(1):43–6.

Savage RR, Kokich VG Sr. Restoration and retention of maxillary anteriors with severe root resorption. J Am Dent Assoc. 2002;133(1):67–71.

Resorption of Impacted Teeth

Glenn T. Sameshima

1 Introduction

There is still much we do not know about how or why teeth become impacted. Maxillary canines in Caucasian populations are more frequently found to be impacted palatally (Strbac et al. 2013), whereas in Asian patients the majority occurs to the buccal. An erupting tooth is destined to resorb the primary tooth as part of the transition from the primary to permanent dentition. Generally, this resorptive process is accomplished by the dental follicle (Becker and Chaushu 2015). Brin et al. (1993) and (Ericson and Kurol 2000) showed dramatically the damage to roots of maxillary lateral incisors caused by adjacent, erupting canine. The apical one-third of the root is the most frequently damaged part of the lateral incisor root as reported in the literature.

Three-dimensional imaging via cone-beam CT has increased our understanding and improved diagnosis to the point where CBCT is standard of care where it is available.

A systematic review of impacted maxillary canines was published in the JADA in 2018 (Schroder et al. 2018). Although the results were inconclusive due to the lack of high-level evidence (no RCTs or case control studies), the authors stated that among their findings was that delayed eruption or *treatment* (italics mine) "may lead to resorption of the adjacent lateral and central incisors." As the quality of 3D imaging improves, evidence is growing that many incisor roots are affected. Hadler-Olsen et al. (2015) found that one-third of all maxillary lateral incisors had non-apical root resorption without an impacted canine; with an impacted adjacent canine, the number nearly doubled. An intriguing finding was found by Becktor et al. (2005). They found a strong association with impacted/ectopic first molars and impacted canines.

G. T. Sameshima (✉)
Advanced Orthodontics, Herman Ostrow School of Dentistry of the University of Southern California, Los Angeles, CA, USA
e-mail: sameshim@usc.edu

© Springer Nature Switzerland AG 2021
G. T. Sameshima (ed.), *Clinical Management of Orthodontic Root Resorption*,
https://doi.org/10.1007/978-3-030-58706-2_10

Current questions for the clinician that remain gray are:

1. Does the dental follicle itself cause damage to the roots of other teeth? It was generally thought that the dental follicle of the erupting canine would inadvertently damage the lateral incisor root but this has not proven to be true as we once thought. Ericson and Kurol (1987a, b, 1988) in a classic series of papers study cast doubt about this theory when they showed that there was no association between the follicle and resorption of the root. Similar investigations over the years have suggested that the follicle may even provide a protective effect and that it is actual physical contact between the crown of the impacted/erupting tooth and the root of the tooth in its pathway. Ericson et al. (2000, 2002) showed using 3D images that there is no association between the follicle and surface root resorption. They theorized that actual contact between the enamel of the canine crown and the root of the lateral incisor is the primary event. This was confirmed by a CBCT study by Alemam et al. (2020) who also found that direct contact between the crown of the canine and root of the incisor was the only significant factor. Dağsuyu et al. (2017) examined the dental follicle width on CBCT images. They concluded that "Our study could not confirm that increased dental follicle width of the maxillary impacted canines exhibited more resorption risk for the adjacent lateral incisors." The study by Rafflenbeul et al. (2019) produced similar findings about dental follicle width and also showed no association between missing or peg laterals and root damage. Regardless of theory, if an erupting canine looks like it is resorbing the lateral incisor root, then orthodontics and surgery must be done to move it away from the root.

2. The second question is regarding cysts. A *dentigerous* or *follicular cyst* was traditionally defined as a dental follicle width (greatest distance between the crown and the follicle on dental 2D radiograph) greater than 2 mm. The distance must be estimated, but the radiolucency surrounding the crown of the maxillary canine in Fig. 1 would appear to qualify. The damage it has produced is evident with the roots of both the maxillary lateral and central incisors that are extensive. However, 3D images have complicated our 2D assessment, and the differential diagnosis of a cyst must include other features such as its size, rate of enlargement, and radiographic appearance in 2D or 3D. According to Becker and Chaushu (2005), the lining of a dentigerous cyst and a normal dental follicle are the same histologically.

3. Which is correct? The canine guidance theory or the genetic theory of maxillary canine eruption? Both remain relevant, and there will probably emerge a combination of both. The clinical and research evidence seem to support both theories (Alqerban et al. 2009).

Case 1

In which the primary canine was NOT extracted (inexplicably, the patient's parent never made the appointment). The sequence of treatment is illustrated in Figs. 2 and 3.

Fig. 1 Typical resorption of the maxillary lateral incisor caused by the eruption of the canine

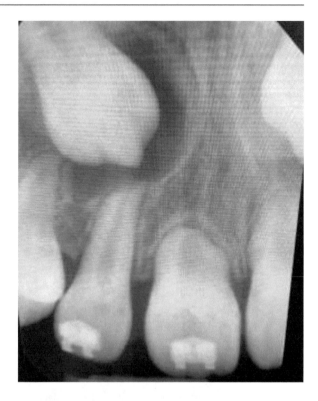

Fig. 2 Initial PAN—note the position of the maxillary right canine. According to the canine guidance theory, if the primary canine is extracted, then the probability of the maxillary canine erupting normally would be increased significantly, although the patient is a 13-year-old male

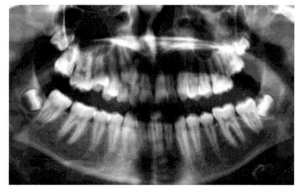

Case 2

11-year-old female. Neg health hx. No trauma? Parents not sure. Hypomineralized enamel generalized. CC: "Tooth won't come in." The progress of the case is described in the legends for Figs. 4, 5, 6, 7, 8, and 9.

Case 3 Large Cysts

We saw how the most affected tooth is the maxillary lateral incisor in a previous chapter. The case is shown in Figs. 10 through 11.

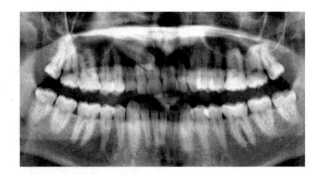

Fig. 3 Six years later at age 19. No treatment was done. The eruption path of the canine has changed dramatically, but fortunately no damage to the roots of the other incisors has occurred yet

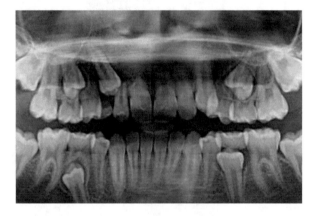

Fig. 4 Initial panoramic image shows late mixed dentition with ectopic eruption of the maxillary right canine. Both maxillary central incisors have short roots, and the right lateral and central incisors appear to have irregular root shape and possible resorption. The orthodontist's treatment plan was to extract the primary right canine immediately and then bond fixed appliances staying in "light wires"

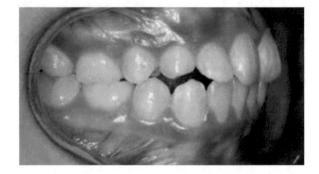

Fig. 5 Initial intraoral image of the right side. Canine bulge is not visible but was palpable by report

Fig. 6 This is a section of the CBCT of Case 3 taken a few months after appliances were placed. The archwire is a round nickel titanium low-force wire

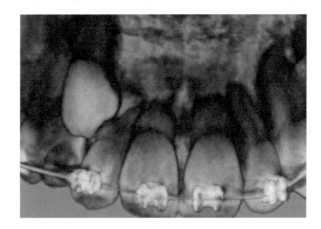

Fig. 7 This is a different view of the same volume shown in the previous figure. Note how close the canine is to the lateral incisor—it is quite likely that the erupting canine crown resorbed the distal side of the lateral incisor

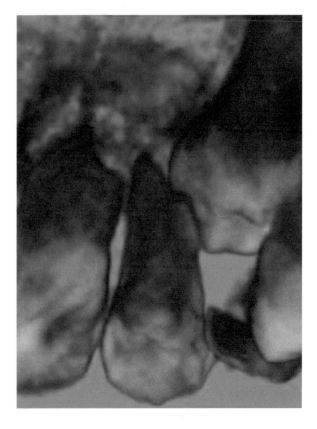

Fig. 8 Source is the same
DICOM file viewed more
occlusally. Notice that the
root length of the right
lateral incisor is the same
as the left lateral incisor,
illustrating the importance
of obtaining a true 3D
view. The maxillary right
central incisor root is
shorter than the left and
has a defect on its
mesial-apical aspect—is
this acquired or
congenital? Without
previous volumetric
images, it is difficult to be
sure, but the clinician
would strongly suspect that
the canine crown was
responsible

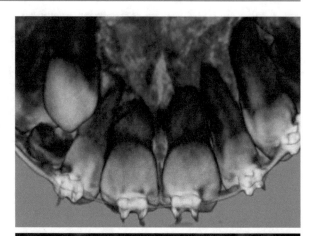

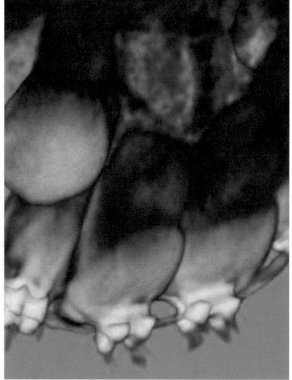

Clinical Case 4

The case in the following figures brings into question the dental follicle/dentigerous
cyst as the cause of root damage to adjacent teeth during the transitional dentition
period. The case is shown in Figs. 12, 13, and 14. The patient was referred by their
family dentist to an orthodontist for evaluation of the missing right "canine" and

Fig. 9 This is another view of the same volume with the hard tissue filter attenuated to show the alveolar bone better. From this image it appears that the canine initially erupted more mesial to the lateral root and then descended more mesially. The lack of bone mesial to the crown is not an artifact, but it will fill in as the tooth erupts into its normal position. Note that this is an initial light nickel titanium round wire of 4 weeks duration and minimal forces have been applied to the incisors

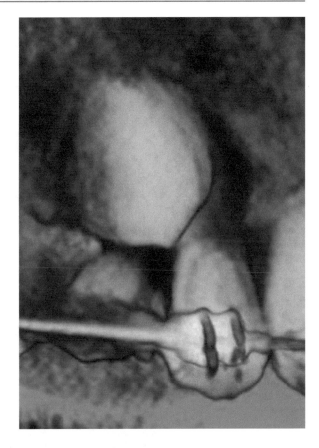

patient parents' concern about spacing. Unfortunately only PANs were available for review. Here is the initial presentation PAN for this healthy, 7-year-old female with a Class I malocclusion of the mixed dentition. Normal overjet and overbite. Negative health history.

The PAN suggests that the impacted maxillary right canine has resorbed the lateral and central incisors. A radiolucent area extends from the crown of the canine to the maxillary right central incisor root apical third. The LCBCT images, however, seem to show less damage. The right lateral incisor root is narrow and more irregular than the left one. The right central incisor has a much shorter and irregular root than the left central. If the canine guidance theory that Juri Kurol proposed long ago is true, then it is likely that the original path of eruption of the right canine was close to the right central incisor root. Regardless, clinical treatment would be the same; surgically exposing the tooth with an open approach, with the force vectors initially moving the crown away from the lateral incisor root.

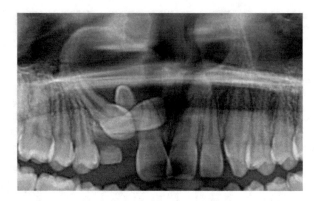

Fig. 10 Pretreatment PAN. Note the large cyst in the maxillary anterior right side causing displacement of the maxillary left lateral incisor and canine. The source of the cyst is the right lateral incisor. A mesiodens is visible on both sides of the maxilla; the right one has been moved by the cyst. The presentation is classic with a unilocular appearance and well-defined pericoronal border. These cysts are normally filled with fluid and appear radiolucent. True cysts can resorb adjacent teeth but rarely do so. Instead the expanding cyst displaces other teeth (especially immature teeth) and can do so in any direction and for a long distance

Fig. 11 Final PAN of the previous case. The lateral incisor and both mesiodens were extracted. Note the dilaceration of the right central incisor caused by the cyst

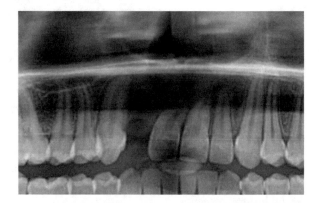

Fig. 12 Initial PAN—note the missing right maxillary lateral incisor. The central incisor roots are short and irregularly shaped. The erupting canines are in normal position

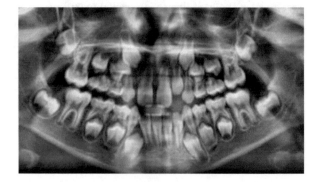

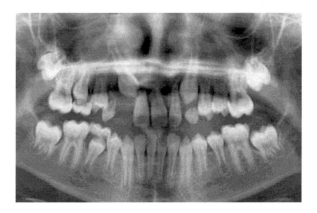

Fig. 13 End of Phase I 2 years later. A maxillary 2 × 4 was used during Phase I to align the existing maxillary incisors. Apical root displacement was negligible. There is moderate irregular root resorption of both maxillary central incisors. The dental follicle is enlarged around the erupting canine. The damage to the LEFT central incisor is difficult to explain

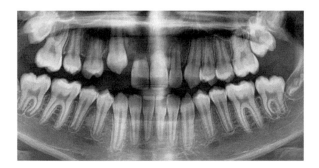

Fig. 14 Two years later. No diagnosis was made of a cyst when the maxillary right primary canine was extracted. The damage to both maxillary central incisors is quite severe. There is a radiolucent area with an ill-defined proximal border that is either a healing prior cyst area or a new cyst

2   Summary and Main Points

Erupting teeth can cause problems, including resorption of the permanent dentition anywhere in the arch, but maxillary canines and mandibular second molars probably cause the most damage. Maxillary canines are intimately related to the lateral incisor during development and eruption. There is plenty of new evidence based on 3D data that have given new insight into the extent of the problem, and it is worse than anyone thought. In 3D there are few maxillary lateral roots that are NOT affected by the neighboring canine. In fact, the amount of damage that some of the lateral incisors sustain is so great that it is surprising that more of them do not have problems later. The surface of the root has a remarkable capacity to heal as evidenced also by studies showing that the root remains vital and functional even when inadvertently assaulted by a mini-implant.

Clinically the dentist should not hesitate to get a 3D view of any tooth that looks like it is not erupting normally on a PAN—should check the other side and the opposite arch for timing. Age and pattern of eruption are also important. Regardless of theory, if the crown of the canine is close to the lateral and the canine root is way more than half developed, then early intervention may be indicated. The dentist must also be suspicious of the presence of a cyst or other pathology if the roots of neighboring teeth are starting to be deflected (dentigerous cyst) or resorbed (e.g., ameloblastoma or OKC). A normal dental follicle can look large on a palatally impacted canine on PAN, still another reason to take a LCBCT to determine precisely the borders of the follicle and the distance from the crown to the root of the lateral incisor. A skilled surgeon or periodontist must be able to expose the tooth especially in the younger patient, and the orthodontist must have good anchorage in place before the surgery.

Does an impacted maxillary canine increase the risk of EARR of the incisors? It might seem logical that even barring radiographic evidence of damage to the adjacent roots that an impacted canine might have an unknown and deleterious effect. An interesting study (Brusveen et al. 2012) dispels this idea. They found no significant difference in EARR between patients with an impacted canine and a control group. Once the offending canine is moved away from the adjacent incisors, there is no increase in risk of EARR during orthodontic treatment.

References

Alemam AA, Abu Alhaija ES, Mortaja K, AlTawachi A. Incisor root resorption associated with palatally displaced maxillary canines: analysis and prediction using discriminant function analysis. Am J Orthod Dentofac Orthop. 2020;157(1):80–90.

Alqerban A, Jacobs R, Lambrechts P, Loozen G, Willems G. Root resorption of the maxillary lateral incisor caused by impacted canine: a literature review. Clin Oral Investig. 2009;13(3):247–55.

Becker A, Chaushu S. Etiology of maxillary canine impaction: a review. Am J Orthod Dentofac Orthop. 2015;148(4):557–67.

Becktor KB, Steiniche K, Kjaer I. Association between ectopic eruption of maxillary canines and first molars. Eur J Orthod. 2005;27(2):186–9.

Brin I, Becker A, Zilberman Y. Resorbed lateral incisors adjacent to impacted canines have normal crown size. Am J Orthod Dentofac Orthop. 1993;104(1):60–6.

Brusveen EM, Brudvik P, Bøe OE, Mavragani M. Apical root resorption of incisors after orthodontic treatment of impacted maxillary canines: a radiographic study. Am J Orthod Dentofac Orthop. 2012;141(4):427–35.

Dağsuyu İM, Okşayan R, Kahraman F, Aydın M, Bayrakdar İŞ, Uğurlu M. The relationship between dental follicle width and maxillary impacted canines' descriptive and resorptive features using cone-beam computed tomography. Biomed Res Int. 2017;2017:5.

Ericson S, Kurol J. Incisor resorption caused by maxillary cuspids: a radiographic study. Angle Orthod. 1987a;57:332–46.

Ericson S, Kurol J. Radiographic examination of ectopically erupting maxillary canines. Am J Orthod Dentofac Orthop. 1987b;91:483–92.

Ericson S, Kurol J. Resorption of maxillary lateral incisors caused by ectopic eruption of the canines. A clinical and radiographic analysis of predisposing factors. Am J Orthod Dentofac Orthop. 1988;94:503–13.

Ericson S, Kurol J. Resorption of incisors after ectopic eruption of maxillary canines: a CT study. Angle Orthod. 2000;70(6):415–23.

Ericson S, Bjerklin K, Falahat B. Does the canine dental follicle cause resorption of permanent incisor roots? A computed tomographic study of erupting maxillary canines. Angle Orthod. 2002;72(2):95–104.

Hadler-Olsen S, Pirttiniemi P, Kerosuo H, Bolstad Limchaichana N, Pesonen P, Kallio-Pulkkinen S, Lähdesmäki R. Root resorptions related to ectopic and normal eruption of maxillary canine teeth—a 3D study. Acta Odontol Scand. 2015;73(8):609–15.

Rafflenbeul F, Gros CI, Lefebvre F, Bahi-Gross S, Maizeray R, Bolender Y. Prevalence and risk factors of root resorption of adjacent teeth in maxillary canine impaction, among untreated children and adolescents. Eur J Orthod. 2019;41(5):447–53.

Schroder AGD, Guariza-Filho O, de Araujo CM, Ruellas AC, Tanaka OM, Porporatti AL. To what extent are impacted canines associated with root resorption of the adjacent tooth?: a systematic review with meta-analysis. J Am Dent Assoc. 2018;149(9):765–77.

Strbac GD, Foltin A, Gahleitner A, Bantleon HP, Watzek G, Bernhart T. The prevalence of root resorption of maxillary incisors caused by impacted maxillary canines. Clin Oral Investig. 2013;17(2):553–64.

Future Directions

Glenn T. Sameshima

1 Introduction

Let us examine one final case. This last case is a well-documented case by Dr. Hideo Nakanishi from Osaka, Japan. The case illustrates many of the points this book has attempted to teach and surprises the reader with an unpredictable ending.

2 Diagnosis and Treatment Plan

This 19-year-old female was referred by her general dentist for evaluation of the impacted left mandibular second molar. The patient is healthy with no history of trauma or harmful oral habits. She has no speech or airway problems. She has a full smile with mild lip strain, and she reports that her front teeth protrude excessively. Cephalometrically she is a skeletal Class I with mild dentoalveolar protrusion. She has moderate crowding with thin gingiva. Oral hygiene is fair. The assumption that the impacted mandibular left molar is a second molar is based on the dental history that no teeth have been extracted. Part of the crown of the tooth is visible in the oral cavity. The mandibular left third molar is assumed to be missing; all other third molars are present. The sequence of treatment images and radiographs are shown in Figs. 1, 2, 3, 4, 5, 6, 7, 8, 9, 10, 11, 12, 13, and 14.

2.1 Initial Orthodontic Records

Initial Orthodontic Records: Figures 1, 2, 3.

G. T. Sameshima (✉)
Advanced Orthodontics, Herman Ostrow School of Dentistry of the University of Southern California, Los Angeles, CA, USA
e-mail: sameshim@usc.edu

© Springer Nature Switzerland AG 2021
G. T. Sameshima (ed.), *Clinical Management of Orthodontic Root Resorption*,
https://doi.org/10.1007/978-3-030-58706-2_11

Fig. 1 Initial
cephalometric film. Patient
has double protrusion with
lip strain and convex
profile. She is interested in
reducing the protrusion.
Zero overjet with open bite
tendency. Mandibular
plane is above average

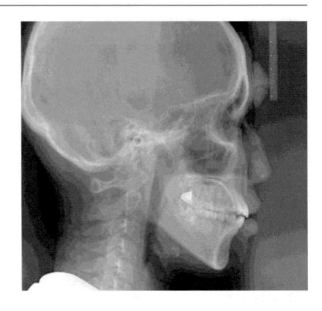

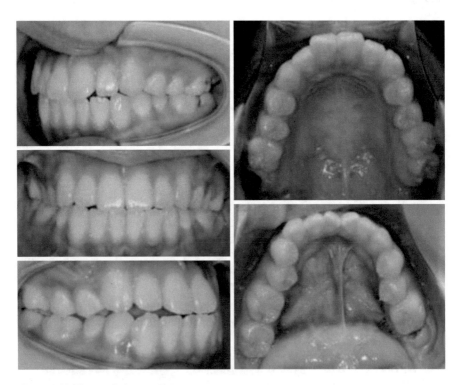

Fig. 2 Initial intraoral photographs

Fig. 2 (continued)

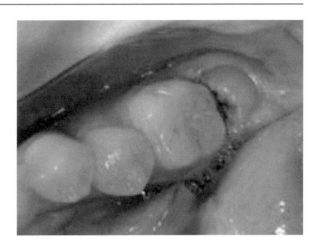

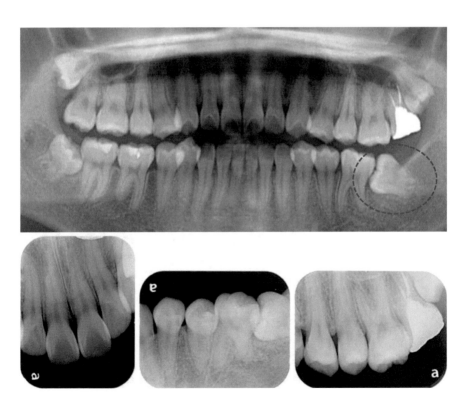

Fig. 3 Initial radiographs. The mandibular left second molar is nearly horizontally impacted, and its root system is difficult to visualize

Fig. 4 The maxillary right second molar was extracted because of poor position and weakened tooth structure. The third molar has already begun to erupt in its place

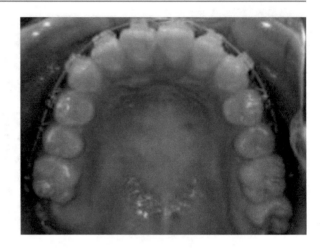

Fig. 5 Five months after appliance placement

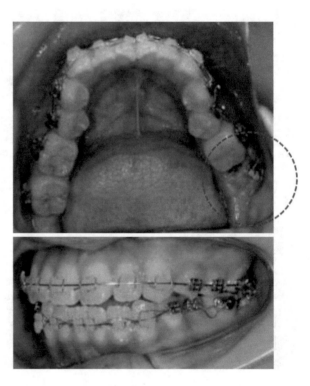

Fig. 6 Nine months

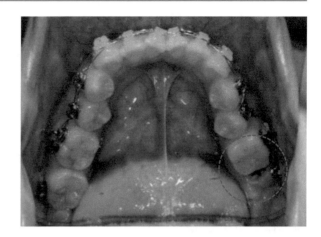

Fig. 7 Progress PAN at 11 months

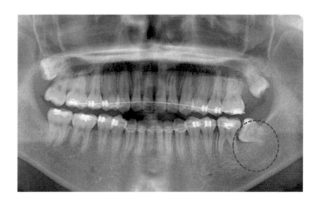

Fig. 8 Separating springs were used to assist in the molar uprighting

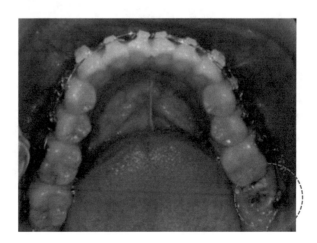

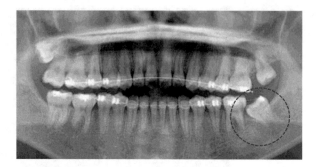

Fig. 9 Progress PAN and image 18 months after appliance placement. The impacted tooth root remains indistinct but appears to be shorter as does the distal root of the adjacent first molar. There is a carious lesion on the distal of the mandibular left first molar. The tooth has tipped distally, but the contact remains gingival

Fig. 10 Progress PAN at 30 months. The mandibular left first molar had successful endodontic therapy. The restorative dentist placed composite over both molars to prevent extrusion of the opposing arch

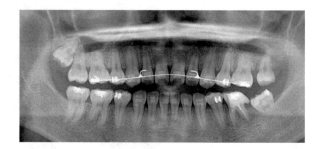

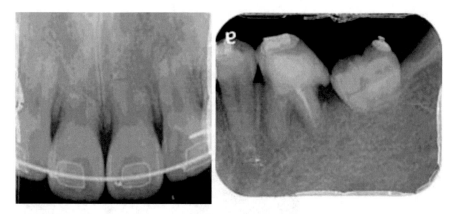

Fig. 11 Periapical radiographs at 30 months of active treatment

Fig. 12 Thirty months progress images—slices from a cone beam CT scan. The 3D image showed there was barely any root structure left in all views

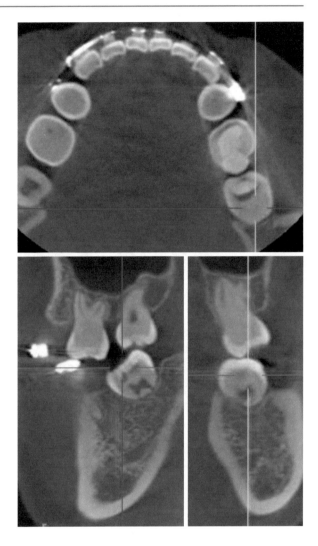

Fig. 13 Final records. See narrative

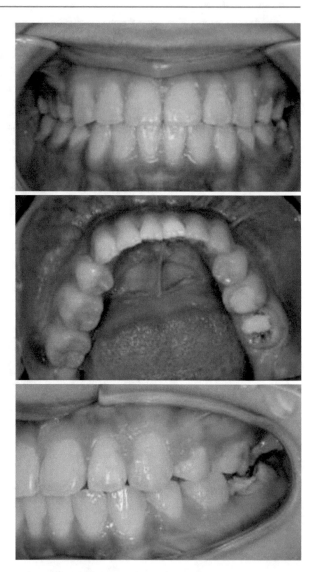

Fig. 14 Two years after appliance removal. Teeth are asymptomatic, and no mobility was found

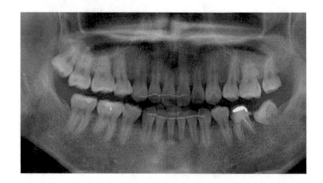

3   Treatment Summary and Conclusions

Treatment sequence: After 1 year, the decision was made to extract first bicuspids for protrusion. The mandibular left second molar proved difficult to upright despite a number of methods. Thirty months after the start of treatment, EARR was discovered and appliances removed shortly thereafter.

Were there any diagnostic risk factors that were present? No. Root shape was normal. Treatment risk factors—long treatment time but not excessive, and apical root displacement—final ceph and tracing not available but case finished in rectangular steel wires to express ideal torque, so the assumption is, yes, palatal root torque. Prognosis? The maxillary right central incisor lost half its root, but the most severely resorbed tooth is clearly the mandibular left second molar. This is unusual for several reasons: (1) mandibular molars rarely have EARR even with intrusion with TADs. (2) Uprighting impacted molars rarely results in EARR if ever. (3) The pattern of EARR seen in this case is bizarre and is atypical of EARR from orthodontic forces. The rate at which the root was lost is astonishing. (4) What will happen to the tooth long term? For now it is being used to prevent the maxillary left molars from overerupting. No mobility or further resorption is present after 20 months. The restorative dentist will decide whether or not to keep the tooth. Conservative dentistry would be to keep the tooth as long as possible to maintain vertical on that side of the mouth.

3.1   Concluding Remarks

The Holy Grail of orthodontic root resorption is prediction and prevention. Ideally the risk factors would have enough power that patients truly at risk would be identified, and then appropriate measures taken. Current scientific advances that will help clear the pathway toward achieving this goal include rapidly improving imaging technology, tests to prove the presence of biological markers of EARR, and sophisticated genetic studies of familial risk. Early detection would help, but until then good progress records are important.

In summary, EARR is considered an unavoidable risk of orthodontic tooth movement. The broad spectrum of magnitude of EARR statistically means that there will be teeth that unpredictably incur severe EARR. This is supported by the fact that severe EARR is relatively uncommon. Clinical management should include recognizing diagnostic and treatment risk factors (such that the treatment goals may require modification), high-quality images, progress records for patients at risk, and an understanding of what to do if severe EARR is found either at progress or at the end of treatment. Educating the patient and referring dentists are equally important. Finally, an extremely important part of this education is informing our dental colleagues that in the long term, there is no increased risk for tooth loss, even for teeth with severe EARR.

Printed in the United States
by Baker & Taylor Publisher Services